BACK

BACK IN SHAPE

A back owner's manual by
Stephen Hochschuler, M.D.
of the **Texas Back Institute**

Back exercise program
demonstrated by
Cory Everson

Edited by
Bob Reznik

Houghton Mifflin Company
Boston

For information about permission to reproduce selections
from this book, write to Permissions, Houghton Mifflin Company,
2 Park Street, Boston, Massachusetts 02108.

Library of Congress Cataloging-in-Publication Data

Hochschuler, Stephen
    Back in Shape : a back owner's manual / Stephen Hochschuler.
        p.   cm.
    Includes index.
    ISBN 0-395-56272-4 (cloth). — ISBN 0-395-56273-2 (paperback)
    1. Backache. 2. Back — Care and hygiene. 3. Self-care, Health.
I.   Title.
RD771.B217H64 1991   90-43031
617.5'6406 — dc20   CIP

Printed in the United States of America

HAD 10 9 8 7 6 5

Book design: Bob Reznik
Medical illustration: Rusty Jones
Photography: Mike Neveux Photography

CONTENTS

It happened to me ...
it could happen to you

I thought the winters at Harvard were rough. Winters in Texas have a flavor all their own. Instead of snow, there are ice storms. Freezing rain glazes the streets, turning cars into 4,000-pound hockey pucks. Fortunately, when there is an ice storm in Texas, the world stops turning and everybody stays home. Except if you're a doctor who is on call.

Even though I've been a spine surgeon now for nearly 15 years, it wasn't until 10 years ago, during a Dallas ice storm, that I had my first real experience with back pain.

The hospital called me. I needed to make it in somehow. I thought my car would get better traction on the ice if I loaded down the rear end. So out in the driveway, cold and shivering, I bent awkwardly over my kid's tricycle to pick up a sack of dry concrete mix. It didn't seem important at the time that I bend my knees. Or that I move the silly tricycle out of the way. I thought I was King Kong.

Lifting the bag of concrete into the trunk was uncomfortable. My back, though sore, seemed okay, and the bag of concrete helped me reach the hospital.

Inside, I bent down to tie my shoe.

I couldn't get up. I felt as though someone had rammed a knife through my back. It took another surgeon, six feet four, to help me straighten out.

The next day was worse. I tried wearing a back corset and taking anti-inflammatories. It wasn't until I was given several facet injections that I started to feel better.

There are mixed blessings to being a spine surgeon and living with a back problem. On the positive side, I can now empathize with what my patients are going through. It's one thing for a doctor to listen to someone moan about his or her back pain. It's another having been there yourself. It's truly indescribable.

I can also understand my patients' fears about treatments. They are noticeably relieved when I tell them that I've had a myelogram, too. And a CT scan. And injections. And I'm the world's biggest chicken.

Yes, there's big relief in knowing your doctor's been there. I see it in their eyes. Misery indeed loves company.

On the down side, though, I have a bulging disc that isn't going to go away. It's there with me for the long haul. For the most part I keep it under control by watching what and how I lift, and by staying in great shape.

There is also a cruel irony in that as a back doctor, I must face unavoidable aspects of the job — like having to stand and bend over for nine hours straight in surgery — which are murder on the back.

I practice what I preach now. I can't remember lifting any more bags of concrete mix in the past 10 years. Certainly none over a tricycle. And when back pain hits me, I use all my home remedies — especially exercise. Sure, it's excruciating at the time. But I know if I stick with it, my back pain will lessen. And it always does.

There are numerous back books on the market written by a variety of doctors. And there is certainly no shortage of general fitness books. Although this book provides great help to the back pain sufferer, it was really written for the person with the healthy back. The bulk of the text emphasizes prevention rather than treatment. Indeed, the single most important message woven into the fabric of the book is that the best way to treat back pain is not after it happens, but before.

Our goal at the Texas Back Institute is simple. We have seen at first hand how back pain can destroy someone's life. It can prevent a person from working. It can prevent a person from loving. For some unfortunate sufferers, it can consume a person's daily existence to the point that even suicide is considered as a way to stop the incessant pain.

In writing this book, we at the Texas Back Institute hope to spare someone from having to live a life handicapped by a severe, debilitating back problem. We hope to enable more people to lead lives not of disability, but ones filled with activity and vitality — all through retirement and their senior years.

Back in Shape is organized in three parts. Part I explains exactly how your back can become injured and the importance of prevention. It also explains who is likely to have a back problem.

Chapter 3, for example, will help you evaluate yourself and your risk of back injury. The fact that you feel no pain now is little indication of your long-term back health. Back pain often occurs not from a single accident, but rather through a process that progresses year after year, until the day when lifting a grocery bag out of the trunk snaps something.

Part II focuses on the best way to get your back in shape and keep it that way, including practical tips to make sports activities and recreation less risky.

Part III goes in depth into what to do if you have an

episode of back pain — something that will happen to most of us no matter how careful we are. This part discusses home remedies, when to see a doctor, and what kind of doctor to see. There is a troubleshooting chapter as well, because often the symptoms of back pain are scary.

Probably the first question that races through a person's mind when back pain happens is "God, will I need surgery?" Chances are overwhelmingly that you won't — if you know a little about your back, and whom to see for professional help. Knowing what each symptom means can lessen the fear and uncertainty considerably, and maybe save you the cost and inconvenience of getting in the car and trucking off to see a doctor.

Through the following chapters, you will learn how to prevent back injury by making your back injury resistant. If you currently experience occasional back pain, which many of us do, there are plenty of first-aid cures, home remedies, exercises, and over-the-counter medications that can be used to manage and shorten the episode when it occurs.

Consider this book as an owner's manual to your back. It's our hope at the Texas Back Institute that this information will ultimately motivate you to be "back in shape," too.

Stephen Hochschuler, M.D.

PART I

The Odds Are Heavily Weighted Against Your Back

1

Back pain:
The price we pay
for walking upright

hances are, most of our ancestors long ago never suffered from back pain. That's because thousands of years ago, our ancestors traversed the savannah with their knuckles dragging along the ground. A cruel fact of nature is that back pain is the price we pay for walking upright.

Fortunately, the spine — even with its intricate series of bones, joints, ligaments and muscles — can be extremely resistant to injury. If it is maintained well. Unfortunately, most Americans are sitting ducks for back pain. In fact, spine research shows that four of every five Americans will experience back pain at some time in their lives.

The more active a person is, the less risk he or she will ever experience back pain. Unlike mechanical components that wear down through the friction of repetitive movement, the body needs motion to retain motion. Simply put, exercise is like WD-40 for the spine; it lubricates the joints and stretches muscles so they are less prone to strain and tearing.

Indeed, many back problems develop because our sedentary lifestyles let our backs get out of condition. Consider the desk-bound executive who lifts nothing heavier than an expensive fountain pen all week long, only to race out to the first tee on Saturday morning, yank the driver out of the bag, and wind up his spine like a human propeller.

When we are young, we can cut corners. We can get away without warming up. But also remember that the young person's muscles are inherently more flexible and resistant to strain. When was the last time you heard of a kid or teenager with back pain?

Muscles and ligaments are like rubber bands. When new, they stretch to great length. But let them get dry and cracked . . . snap! The rubber band tears instead of stretches.

Are you at risk for back pain?

Back pain is a working person's problem in that the risk of having it escalates in the middle years — from ages 30 to 55 — with both men and women suffering equally. It is truly an equal opportunity disease, affecting individuals without regard to race, occupation, religion, or personal wealth. Each year the Texas Back Institute sees thousands of people from across the United States, from the 240-pound roughneck oil rigger of West Texas with the back of Atlas, to a country singer like Willie Nelson, who probably heaves nothing heavier than a guitar case or a set of golf clubs into the trunk of his car.

The stories we hear of how patients received their back injuries are no less intriguing. We stopped trying to guess a long time ago. Perhaps the winner in our annual contest of the most bizarre back injury is professional golfer Lee Trevino.

Golf is a wicked sport for the spine. The coiling, the torque . . . we weren't surprised that he was injured on a golf course.

Guess again?

Sure enough, Trevino did injure his back while playing

golf. During the Western Open, a storm rolled over the golf course, disrupting play. Trevino took off his golf spikes, opened his umbrella, and leaned against his golf bag. A lightning bolt streaked down from the heavens and skimmed along the surface of a nearby lake over to the golf bag, up the metal shafts of his golf clubs, and into Lee's back, sending voltage up his spine and out through his shoulder. Miraculously, he survived, but with excruciating back pain as a lifetime calling card from Mother Nature. Believe it. Back pain will get you, too.

Trevino does things a lot differently now. Even with his back problem, he is still top-rated as a tour professional, although we tell him to hit fewer practice balls per training session and to keep up his daily back exercises. And if you're watching a golf tournament on television and the sky begins to darken menacingly, you'll notice he is the first one beating a path for the clubhouse.

Certain occupations have higher risk of back pain. Garbage collectors, for example, are at the highest possible risk of having an on-the-job back injury because they must repeatedly perform the most difficult motion for the spine: bending, lifting, and then twisting with a load that is held away from the body. Combine that motion with tossing a heavy garbage bag several feet forward into the back of a moving truck, and you can see why each year one of every 10 garbage collectors has an on-the-job back injury.

Such statistics can be misleading, however, in that they show who is most likely to make an on-the-job back injury claim. If you are a secretary or office worker, don't assume you are at low risk for a back injury. You may in fact be at higher risk for an off-hours back injury. Studies done at the Texas Back Institute show that 75 percent of all back injuries happen away from work.

Who is more at risk for an off-hours back injury? The garbage collector who is up at five in the morning Monday through Friday to train for the year when the 50-pound plastic sack heave becomes a sanctioned Olympic event? Or the guy who pushes a pencil at his job five days a week, then goes out on the weekend to tote 50-pound bags of fertilizer around the yard, and then plays five sets of killer tennis later that afternoon?

In reality, the garbage collector's back muscles are likely to be so strong that unless he's into lifting Sherman tanks in his off hours, he's ready for anything the weekend throws at him. The persons at most risk for back injury are those who are most inactive. Sure, certain occupations can be tough on the back. But having a sedentary desk job during the week is a setup for back injury. Because who sits around on the weekend? Nah, we head for the lake, strap a couple of boards to the bottom of our feet, and let a boat drag us around at the end of a rope until our spines get the full jackhammer treatment. We crawl back into the boat three inches shorter than when we started. Now that's what weekends are all about. Get the picture?

Back pain is a gradual disease

Another thing to consider is that although many back problems end up as on-the-job injuries, they don't necessarily start there.

The human back has to be conditioned for all the activities that you intend to throw at it, whether at work or at play. Too much tennis on Sunday can set you up for a back strain when you lift a small box of computer paper Monday morning. Technically, the strain you suffer when lifting the box qualifies as an on-the-job back injury and for worker's compensation benefits. But really, what caused the back injury?

Many doctors avoid using the term *back injury* simply because it implies trauma, and that back pain occurs all of a sudden at a specific time and place. But many studies have shown that low back pain is in fact gradual in 60 percent of cases.

Back problems too often occur not from traumatic falls from ladders at work, but from lifting something that should have been within people's normal capabilities. If they were in shape. If they were warmed up. If they used proper lifting form. Or if the job were designed in a way to help rather than abuse the back.

Employers are recognizing that in an era of sky-high worker's compensation premiums, investing in the prevention of back injury now makes good economic sense. Consequently, more plants are targeting high-injury jobs and redesigning them to make them easier on the back. Old chairs are being replaced with ergonomically designed chairs that support the low back and make long periods of sitting easier. At last, awareness of the benefits of prevention are hitting the work place.

The price tag of back pain

By some estimates, Americans spend more than $16 billion in their quest for relief from back pain. At any given time, 31 million Americans — about one in eight people — will have low back pain, according to Liberty Mutual Insurance Company.

Why is Liberty Mutual so concerned? Because as the largest single payer of worker's compensation claims in the United States, Liberty Mutual pays out $1 million every working day to cover low back pain claims by injured workers. Not surprisingly, back pain is one of the most common, most expensive, and most litigious of on-the-job injuries. Common doesn't necessarily mean cheap, however. The National Council on Compensation Insurance reports that the cost of the average back strain or sprain is nearly $6,000.

Fortunately, for most victims back injury is usually minor and will often go away on its own. For others, the process of healing can be helped with a combination of rest, therapy, and sometimes aspirin. Only a small percentage of individuals have truly serious back problems, which consume disproportionate amounts of money for treatment. Liberty Mutual estimates that 20 percent of back pain cases account for 80 percent of the costs.

On the low end, a simple back strain can be treated with 50 cents' worth of aspirin. On the high end, for a serious back injury the sky is the limit. The National Council on Compensation Insurance notes that the average cost to treat a herniated disc, for example, is nearly $23,500. Where does the money go? About one-third goes to doctors for medical care. Another third goes to hospitals. The last third goes to the injured person and his or her attorney in the form of disability payments and settlements.

Back pain is an unwelcome visitor. It comes without warning, it takes too long to leave, and once it knows your address it returns too frequently.

If you have back pain, there are ways to keep it at a distance. If you don't have back pain, consider yourself lucky — for the time being — because the odds are still overwhelming. Except maybe for the person who is back in shape.

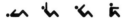

2

What causes back pain?

The human spine is a wondrous piece of human architecture — a series of shock-absorbing discs and bony vertebrae stacked neatly on one another like cups and saucers. Woven into the center of this stack is the spinal cord, the main highway of nerves which transports sensations and commands between the brain and the body.

Around this tower of vertebrae are muscles that serve as guy wires, keeping everything in place, even under incredible stress. Designed into the structure is an automatic internal lubrication system to combat friction and wear and a fail-safe mechanism to prevent overrotation and excessive twisting.

The perfect spine appears straight and upright from the back or front view, but a side view reveals that it is actually not straight at all. In fact, the perfect spine forms an S shape with a slight curve in the low back and another near the neck. The curves allow the spine to carry great body weight, as well as generate incredible lifting force.

The spine, when you analyze it fully, is an engineering masterpiece. It is strong yet flexible. It can lift tremendous amounts of weight but is a comparatively light component of our bodies. It has a remarkable ability to remain healthy and fix itself. It is only after an attack of back pain that we realize that the structure can send forth confusing signals from its abundant set of nerves.

To understand why back pain happens and how it can be prevented, you need to know a little bit about how the spine works.

Vertebrae: The building blocks of the spine

If the spine were composed of a single bone, consider how different your body would be. You would only be able to bend at the waist. And to see to the side, you would have to turn your entire body.

Instead of a one-piece bone, the spine is composed of 25 separate bones called vertebrae. (A single bone unit is

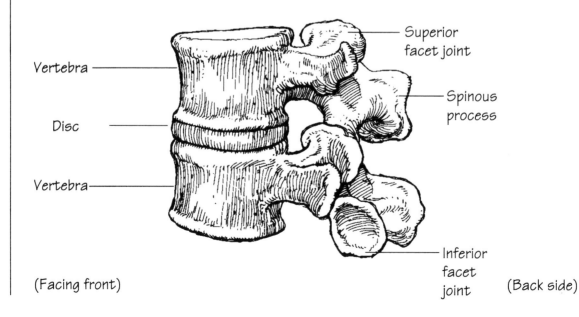

Vertebra

Disc

Vertebra

Superior facet joint

Spinous process

Inferior facet joint

(Facing front)   (Back side)

called a vertebra.) Each bone is round and about an inch in height. At the back of each bone are two prongs that serve as hinges, connecting a vertebra to the one above and the one below. The mechanism allows for the spine to twist right and left, up and down.

Imagine all these bones stacked on top of one another. Now imagine what would happen if you jumped up and down. The force might crack, or fracture, these bones as they hit together. Or over time, just the friction of all the movement might wear the bony surfaces. Fortunately, there are shock absorbers built into the system in the form of discs.

Discs: Jelly doughnuts in the back

The disc itself is made up of an inner spongy portion called the nucleus pulposus and an outer, harder ring of fibrous tissue called the annulus fibrosis. The outer rings of the

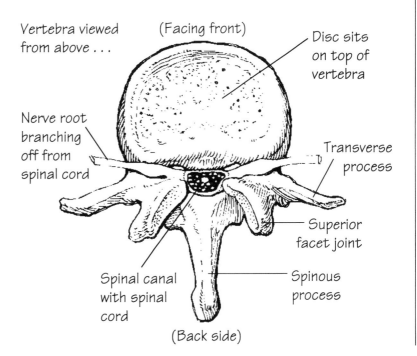

Vertebra viewed from above . . .

(Facing front)

Disc sits on top of vertebra

Nerve root branching off from spinal cord

Transverse process

Superior facet joint

Spinal canal with spinal cord

Spinous process

(Back side)

disc resemble the rings of a tree.

Typically, the discs can take a lot of abuse from us without complaining. Unfortunately, that's not necessarily good, because we assume we aren't hurting our backs when in some cases we can be doing permanent damage. For example, the jelly center of the doughnut can be continually squashed, breaking through more and more outer disc rings. Still, we may not feel any pain, and may continue with our bad posture and bad lifting habits. Eventually, an outer wall may bulge out and put pressure on a nearby nerve where it connects to the spinal cord. That's when we get the first message loud and clear from the disc: back pain.

If we really put pressure on an already weakened disc by lifting something heavy without strong enough back muscles to share the load, we can rupture, or herniate, the disc. A herniated disc is sometimes erroneously referred to as a "slipped disc," implying that the disc has slipped out of place and can be deftly manipulated back into its proper place by a doctor. In reality, there is no such thing as a slipped disc. Discs can't slip because they are attached by connective tissue to vertebrae above and below. When a disc herniates, the jelly center squirts out of the disc wall to put pressure on nearby nerves. Hold on to your hat when this happens, because your disc will definitely let you know you did something wrong.

It is important to note that although the disc can be self-lubricating and injury resistant, it cannot repair itself when torn. Consequently, while pain can be relieved, the damage done to a disc can be permanent and has real consequences — for life.

Worse, age is not on our side because blood supply to the disc itself stops around the age of 20. The disc can go into a state of slow degeneration where it can become drier, flatter, and more susceptible to herniation as we grow older. By doing flexibility and aerobic exercises, we help the disc to lubricate itself as well as stay healthy from the increased blood flow to the areas surrounding the disc space.

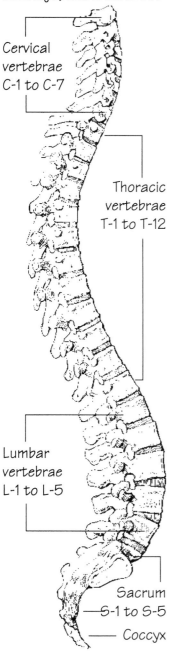

The back, when viewed sideways, has a curve . . .

Cervical vertebrae C-1 to C-7

Thoracic vertebrae T-1 to T-12

Lumbar vertebrae L-1 to L-5

Sacrum S-1 to S-5

Coccyx

Facet joints

Take your hand and reach around to the center of your back. Run your fingers down toward the low back. Those bony projections you feel through the skin are called the spinous process.

On either side of the spinous process are facet joints, which serve as a hinge between the vertebra above and the one below. The function of each facet joint is to guide, direct, and limit the movement of the spine. Unlike the vertebral body, which is a sturdy block of bone, the facet joints are not designed to carry excessive body weight. We cringe when we see people lifting heavy loads in hyperextended, or arched back, position.

Each facet joint is surrounded by a capsule of connective tissue. This capsule secretes a lubricating substance called synovial fluid, which helps the hinges of the back move smoothly and without friction. Keeping all the facet joints firmly in place is a series of ligaments.

Lifting or straining with an arched back puts abnormal stress on the facet joints which can in turn fracture or inflame the joint capsules. Either way, the result is back pain.

The spine from top to bottom:
The cervical, thoracic, and lumbar lingo

As in any other field of medicine, physicians have special terms for various components of the spine. Understanding the terms will make it easier to talk with your back doctor. Physicians categorize the spine into three separate sections.

The cervical spine includes the top seven vertebrae in the neck area, which are labeled C-1 through C-7, top to bottom. The neck bones are small and fragile and move freely, allowing our heads to turn and see around us while our bodies remain stationary. The vertebrae in the neck are not as large or strong as vertebrae in the trunk area. The cervical spine is important because it protects the spinal cord where it

The back, when viewed from behind,
should appear straight . . .

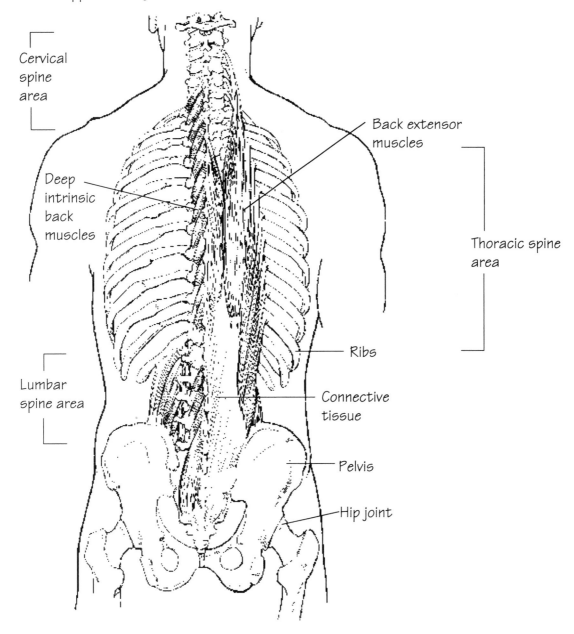

Cervical
spine
area

Back extensor
muscles

Deep
intrinsic
back
muscles

Thoracic spine
area

Ribs

Lumbar
spine area

Connective
tissue

Pelvis

Hip joint

attaches to the brain. Each summer there are hundreds of cases of individuals diving into shallow water, hitting bottom, and fracturing vertebrae and the spinal cord in the neck area. Interrupting the flow of nerve impulses in this area can cause a tragic result: paralysis from the neck down.

Below the cervical vertebrae is the thoracic spine, also called the upper back. The thoracic area of the spine includes 12 vertebrae labeled from T-1 (top) to T-12 (bottom). The vertebrae of the middle and upper back are slightly larger and less mobile than the others, with places where the twelve pairs of ribs connect on either side.

Below the thoracic spine are the five vertebrae that compose the infamous lumbar spine, or low back. These are labeled L-1 through L-5, top to bottom. We'll talk a lot about this area later.

At the bottom of the spine is a large solid bone called the sacrum. It's held tightly between the iliac bones of the pelvis on either side, which together form the sacroiliac joints.

The coccyx (pronounced "cock six") is the bottom-most tip of the human spine, and resembles a small bony finger. It's all we have left of the tail we inherited from the monkeys and apes.

Some interesting party trivia: Did you know that some people have five small bones in their coccyx area, whereas others have only four? If you ever need X rays of your low back, ask the doctor to count the bones in your coccyx. If you have five, maybe you can brag to your friends about being a more direct descendant of King Kong.

When stacked atop one another, the vertebrae line up, forming a hollow tube inside the spine called the spinal canal, which houses and protects the spinal cord.

Muscles: The guy wires around the tower

It's estimated that most back pain is caused by soft tissue injury, such as muscle strain. There are two main muscle groups that make or break the back: extensors and flexors.

Visualize a big rubber band attached at the top to your chest and at the bottom below your belly button. Visualize another the same length on your back. Picture what would happen to the rubber bands when you bent over to pick something up. The rubber band in back has a tough job of straightening you up, as well as all the weight your arms are holding. And if your arms are holding something out in front of the body, the lifting strain increases dramatically.

The extensor muscles lie in the center of the back and enable us to straighten up and lift things. Rather than one thick rubber band, the back muscles are composed of a myriad of small muscles working together. They attach to the back part of the spine and pass from one vertebra to another. Each individual muscle, however, spans only two or three vertebrae. As you can imagine, there is a lot of teamwork among the extensor muscles.

The flexor muscles, conversely, are in front and include all the abdominal muscles. The flexor muscles enable us to bend forward. Flexors are also important during lifting because of oblique abdominal muscles, which go sideways and anchor to the back. These abdominals also help control the amount of arch or swayback (lordosis) in the low back. They begin at the lower edge of the rib cage and breastbone and pass down in front of the stomach and attach to the pelvis. The gluteal, or buttock, muscles begin at the top of each side of the pelvis in the back, pass down behind the hip, and attach to the top of the leg bone (femur). The latissimus dorsi muscles, which attach to the pelvis and spine through a thick ligament, similarly stabilize the pelvic area. All these individual muscles work closely with the abdominal muscles in controlling the position of the pelvis and providing support for the spine.

To illustrate the importance of being in good physical shape, consider what happens to the spine when stomach muscles are poorly toned. Men with big beer bellies are classic examples of how the stomach can pull the trunk forward out of alignment. This disalignment puts even greater strain on the spine when lifting. Similarly, it's common for pregnant women to suffer from sporadic back pain during the latter months of pregnancy.

Thigh, or quadricep, muscles are the body's powerhouse muscles capable of generating great explosive force. The stronger a person's legs, the less load transmitted to the spine. The leg muscles are the best possible place to shift the burden of lifting because back muscles are more prone to "binding up," or going into a spasm, under heavy loads.

The stomach flexor muscle group help the back bend and lift . . .

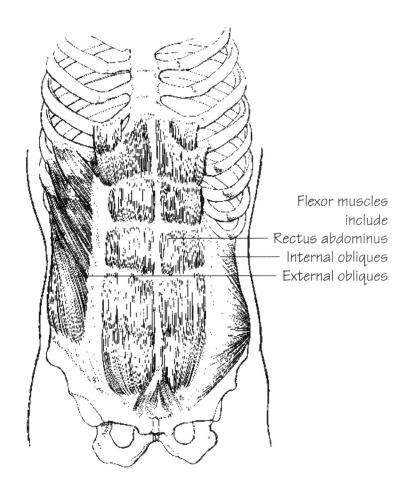

Flexor muscles
include
Rectus abdominus
Internal obliques
External obliques

What happens when the muscles that support our posture don't do their jobs? The ligaments must then take over to hold the body up. If the ligaments do double-duty for long periods of time, they will stretch and lose their ability to maintain our upright posture. The natural spinal curves may then increase an excessive amount, which encourages even more problems.

As you can see, all of the structures in the spine — vertebrae, discs, facet joints, ligaments, muscles and nerves — together make the healthy back a workhorse.

The three main sources of back pain: Muscles, discs, and joints

In a structure as intricate as the spine, a lot can go wrong. A problem at any one of the joints can disrupt and cripple the whole back. Scoliosis, or curvature of the spine, is one common problem. Tumors can also grow in the spinal column. In the case of inflammatory arthritis, the cushioning discs lose their sponginess and cease to insulate the vertebrae.

Although the causes of back pain are varied, 80 percent of cases can be traced to one of three causes:

Muscle strain

In normal operation, the muscles of the back contract and relax as the back moves. But sometimes, under strain, an out-of-shape muscle can spasm, tensing up to the point that it becomes a hard lump. What we feel is a sharp pain, what is often called a charley horse.

A muscle can cramp up for a variety of reasons, including wear and overuse, such as in tennis elbow. Or it can cramp because of a facet joint problem. Even emotional stress can do it.

Fortunately, with rest, ice, and a few aspirins, the pain will often subside. But muscles have a memory, and can strain again if not strengthened and made more resilient.

Herniated discs

The second source of back pain can be traced to a bulging or herniated disc that puts pressure on a nearby spinal nerve. Wear and tear or age of the disc may lead to a deterioration of the disc's outer walls. This deterioration may allow the walls to bulge more than they normally would under stress. The disc is elastic enough to bulge to some degree, but it may bulge to a greater degree if it has deteriorated. If it is bulging to a significant degree it can press on nerve roots or the spinal cord, causing irritation of those structures. If the disc walls deteriorate enough, or if the disc receives additional strain in the form of a sudden, heavy lift, the jelly center can squirt out through the walls, putting pressure on nearby nerves. Worse, if the jelly breaks loose into a free-floating fragment, it can migrate to other positions outside the disc.

Unlike a sore knee or elbow, the spine is like a complex electrical circuit with main lines branching off into smaller ones. Consequently, finding the short can be tough. One common complication of disc-related back pain is that it can create pain that travels into other parts of the body. Because the nerve roots branching off from the spinal cord act as telegraph lines to other parts of the body, pain and irritation can be communicated there as well. We may feel pain that radiates down

When a disc herniates, the jelly center presses against and irritates nearby nerves . . .

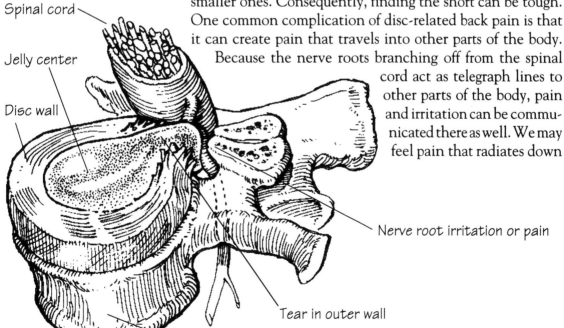

Spinal cord

Jelly center

Disc wall

Nerve root irritation or pain

Tear in outer wall

Vertebra

into a shoulder or arm, but the cause of the pain lies a relatively great distance away in a bulging or herniated disc in the neck. In the low back, similarly, nerves bundle up to form the sciatic nerve, which travels down the back of the leg. Again, leg pain is a common by-product of back problems.

Treating the symptoms of back pain doesn't accomplish anything if the cause of the problem is not identified and treated. And the signal your brain is receiving provides only a clue as to where to look for the central cause of your back pain.

Facet joints

Facet joints should line up precisely with those above and below, enabling the back to twist and bend with little friction among the bones. When a facet joint is sprained by a sudden jerk or twist, it can cause pain much like a knee joint sprain. Likewise, if the joint capsules lose their lubrication and become rough, the common result is back pain.

Probably the single most troublesome part of the spine — regardless of whether it is a muscle, disc, or facet joint problem — is the lumbar spine, or low back area. It is usually the area of the spine which receives the most stress and strain. As a result, more spine problems occur in the lumbar region than anywhere else.

Other causes of back problems

Most back problems fit into the above categories, but there are several other less common causes of back pain that deserve mentioning.

Lordosis and kyphosis

Picture a profile of a person's body as he stands facing to the left. Lordosis refers to the forward curve of the lumbar spine when viewed from the side, kyphosis to the backward curve of the thoracic spine.

Excess lordosis, or inward curve, may be caused by a

congenital defect, that is, one present at birth, or a disease related to certain elements of the spine. In some cases it may be a postural problem, such as in people who have large, protruding abdomens. Regardless of the cause, the result is that the curve can put stress on the facet joints. Straightening of the lumbar spine to remove the lordotic curve may itself cause pain by placing new pressure on the disc spaces. Kyphosis at that level may indicate muscle spasms or even fractures of the vertebral bodies within the lower lumbar spine.

Maintaining the normal and natural curve of the spine through good posture is the best way to distribute the load on the spine evenly among all the structures that are designed to carry it.

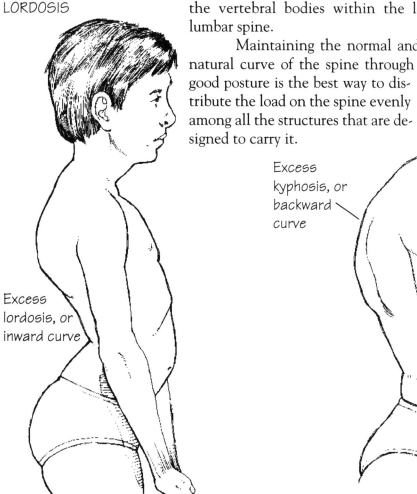

LORDOSIS

Excess
lordosis, or
inward curve

Excess
kyphosis, or
backward
curve

KYPHOSIS

Spinal stenosis

Have you ever gotten a ring stuck on your finger? First it seemed tight. Then as a reaction to the ring, your finger swelled, making the ring even tighter. Luckily, you were able to cut the ring off.

Spinal stenosis, similarly, refers to a shrinking of the spinal canal. A reduction in the size of the spinal canal can be congenital or it can be developmental, meaning it occurs as the body grows and ages.

Stenosis can be caused by arthritis, surgery, an injury, or in some cases a change in posture. As the spinal canal shrinks, there is less and less room for the spinal cord and nerves to move freely. Consequently, they can be irritated and inflamed and swell to a larger size, which makes the problem even worse. Spinal stenosis is a difficult problem to treat conservatively and sometimes requires surgery to increase the size of the spinal canal.

Scoliosis

Scoliosis is a condition in which the spine is curved sideways. As we noted, the normal spine has slight natural curves. But when viewed from the front or behind, it should appear straight.

For some people, however, the spine doesn't develop correctly as they grow up. Instead of the S curve growing straight, it twists perversely like a corkscrew. This abnormal spinal development can show itself first as a walking or posture problem, or as a hump in a person's back.

Experts aren't sure why scoliosis happens. It's not a birth defect because in most cases the person isn't born with the problem. Except for infantile scoliosis, which is rare, scoliosis often doesn't appear until age 10 — during the growth spurt of adolescence. A current theory is that there might be an inherited predisposition for asymmetrical, or

A vertebra and spinal canal viewed from above . . .

(Front)

Vertebra

Spinal canal

Stenosis: When the spinal canal shrinks it can crimp the spinal cord, causing irritation or pain . . .

(Back)

Scoliosis: The spine begins to twist as it grows, resembling a bent corkscrew . . .

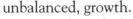

unbalanced, growth.

Relatively few patients with scoliosis require surgery. The problem is more serious for children or teenagers whose spines begin to curve too much during their growth spurts. Once teenagers reach their adult height, if the curve is not severe it will usually not get worse. Curves of greater than 30 degrees, however, may in fact get worse, needing surgery to prevent serious or life-threatening internal complications. Mild curves can sometimes be the cause of back pain. An adult with scoliosis may have an occasional backache more often than a person without scoliosis. In any event, back pain from mild scoliosis can often be lessened with back strengthening exercises. (See Chapter 12 for more information on how scoliosis can be treated.)

Spondylolysis and spondylolisthesis

Spondylolysis refers to a defect in a specific part of the facet joint called the pars interarticularis. This defect can cause instability in the vertebra, much like a loose hinge on a door.

Over time, with ongoing stresses, the ligaments and muscles that help hold the vertebral body in place may become overworked and stretched. As a result, the entire vertebral body can slide forward, which can cause

Spondylolysis: When a defect in the facet joint causes instability . . .

Spondylolisthesis: When the defect allows the vertebra to slide forward . . .

nerves to be pinched, causing pain. This sliding of the vertebral body is called spondylolisthesis. Both spondylolysis and spondylolisthesis can be present at birth or occur through an injury.

Mild cases of spondylolysis and spondylolisthesis usually cause no pain at all. Indeed, it is often discovered incidentally when a person has a preemployment examination or X rays of the back for an unrelated reason.

When spondylolysis and spondylolisthesis cause pain, it is usually treated by strengthening back muscles and avoiding heavy lifting. If that treatment is unsuccessful, a spine surgeon can use a bone graft to fuse the loose vertebrae surgically and keep them from sliding out of place.

Whiplash

Whiplash, as the word graphically implies, occurs when the head and neck are jerked violently. This injury usually occurs from rapid deceleration, as in a head-on or rear-end car collision.

As the head is thrown forward, the muscles in the back of the neck are stretched rapidly. This rapid stretching causes receptors in the muscles and tendons to fire, causing a reflex action that contracts these muscles violently, snapping the head backward. The damage is done either by the rapid stretching or when the head snaps backward with the contraction of the cervical muscles.

The classical definition of whiplash is: "partial dislocation or subluxation of the cervical vertebral facet joints, damaging the capsule of the facet and the adjacent soft tissues."

Amazingly, however, it is relatively rare for whiplash injury to herniate a cervical disc. It is even more rare for it to actually fracture a cervical vertebra. It can strain or even tear ligaments or muscles, which can be treated and rehabilitated in the same manner as any other neck or back injury.

Unfortunately, whiplash is a term that has come to

enjoy a secondary meaning, perhaps because it is often misused by some lawyers who automatically see green when they hear the word. In reality, the whiplash motion causes neck injury not unlike other neck injuries. As such, most uncomplicated neck injuries can be treated successfully. Too often, however, whiplash becomes complicated because sufferers begin to think they have a special type of neck injury, one that is more serious than others and that is less prone to recovery. They have programmed themselves for failure and to expect pain rather than concentrating on recovery, as would others with a neck strain.

In summary, the best way to understand whiplash is to remember it only as the manner in which an injury happened rather than a specific and severe type of injury, which it often isn't. Suppose you hurt your back by tossing a heavy rock. Would you then brag to your friends you have "rocktoss"? Gee, is that worse than "slipandfall"?

If your neck is injured in a car accident, find out if a disc is damaged, if ligaments are strained or torn, or if muscles need rebuilding. Then dispense with any special badges for your injury and get on with your recovery.

Coccygeal pain

As the term implies, coccygeal pain refers to pain emanating from the coccyx, or bottom of the spine. Coccygeal pain is sometimes referred to as coccydynia. The cause of this problem is sometimes vague and difficult to establish. One of the more common causes of coccydynia is falling and hitting the tail bone on the floor or the stairs. Also, since the tail bone is the focus of pressure in a sitting posture, it can become irritated. Such pain can be annoying and difficult to get rid of, but it is rarely a serious problem that requires drastic intervention. It is usually treated by removing pressure on the coccyx by sitting on a cushion that displaces some of the body's weight onto the buttocks and legs. It can also be treated with anti-inflammatory medicine, such as aspirin or ibuprofen. If that doesn't work, pain can be relieved by injecting cortisone around the coccyx. Even so, the pain can return without reason. Interestingly, such pain can also be related to psychological stress.

Arthritis

Arthritis is a disease that causes joints to become painfully inflamed, restricting their range of motion. Some people suffer from muscle spasm as well. Although there are exceptions, arthritis usually affects older adults.

Arthritis is probably most noticeable when it swells finger joints, often causing the fingers to grow crooked. In the back, arthritis can dramatically restrict the range of motion and cause great pain.

Traditionally, arthritis has been treated with aspirin and inactivity like bed rest. Recently, however, exercise has been recommended more and more by arthritis experts. Aerobic exercise for building cardiovascular strength and specific exercises that strengthen muscles around afflicted joints are suggested. Because exercise can heighten existing pain, it is important that the arthritis sufferer consult a physician and a physical therapist before starting any exercises.

Osteoporosis

Osteoporosis, as the name implies, is a disease that causes the bones to become porous and brittle. The result is that they can easily fracture. Like arthritis, osteoporosis tends to affect older adults. Women especially are the prime target of this disease. Some estimates note that 50 percent of women over the age of 80 have evidence of vertebral fractures.

Dietary supplements such as increased calcium have been recommended in the past to slow the loss of bone mass. Estrogen has also shown some ability to slow the progression of osteoporosis.

Persons with osteoporosis are at extremely high risk for back problems as the spinal vertebrae become prone to fracture and degeneration.

As with arthritis, exercise is being scrutinized as a way to slow bone decay. Several studies have shown that physical inactivity to the point of weightlessness or immobilization can lead to a decrease in bone mineral density. These same studies show that greater physical activity, as seen in athletes, can increase bone density. However, women whose periods stop because of too much exercise face increased risk of osteoporosis.

Those with osteoporosis should consult a physician before embarking on any type of exercise program, including the exercises shown in this book.

Back pain caused by poor posture

Both at home and at work, we get into positions — whether bending, twisting, sitting or standing — that can trigger simple back pain.

Briefly, the pressure placed on the discs in the spine changes as the position, or posture, of the spine changes. The least possible strain is placed on our backs, and the intervertebral discs, when we're lying down — flat on our backs. No surprise. But did you know that as soon as we stand up, the pressure on the discs increases to three times what is was lying down? Sitting is even greater: four times the pressure of lying down.

When we lift a box of medium weight, the pressure on the discs increases to more than five times what it was lying down. That's assuming we lift it with perfect body mechanics. Using improper body mechanics, like when we bend over at the waist instead of bending at the knees, the pressure on our discs is increased 10 times!

Besides increasing disc pressure, poor posture stretches the ligaments. A good example of this occurs when a worker has to stay hunched over a workbench or factory assembly line. Also, if we lift without warming up, we are not as flexible as we might be, which similarly increases the likelihood of muscle and ligament strain.

In summary, the effects of poor posture include

- increased risk of pressure on the discs, nerves, and facet joints
- poor mechanical leverage for the spinal structure when lifting
- strain to the muscles and ligaments of the back, leading to fatigue

Pain is different for different people

What is causing your back pain? As you can see, because of the complexity of the spine, often there are no quick answers. In some cases, diagnosing a back problem is like throwing a metal wrench into the circuitry of a computer and then asking a technician to determine which wires have shorted out.

Aside from the complex nature of the spine, people themselves have different thresholds of pain. This pain threshold can be related to cultural factors, personality traits, and even social and economic factors.

Furthermore, because a backache can cause loss of a job, it is common for a person's psychological state to be affected as well. Instead of just having back pain to worry about, a myriad of associated life problems arise: "Who's going to pay the bills now that I can't work? Can I find another job? Will I ever work again? I'm not a good provider . . . does my wife still love me?" Boom, throw a case of depression on top of back pain.

Moreover, if a person has had back pain over a long period of time without seeking proper care, chances are he or she may unknowingly have become drug dependent from trying to mask the pain without fixing the underlying cause. Now try sorting out an addiction problem.

Compound all this with the fact that pain in and of itself is difficult to define and measure, and you can see why back pain makes doctors pull their hair out. It can be just too darn frustrating. Not surprisingly, some doctors even refuse to see back pain patients.

By virtue of their training, all doctors want to help a patient who is suffering. It is extremely frustrating for them when they cannot relieve a person's pain. Too often, back surgery is considered as the next step for relieving pain, only because a particular doctor has no other alternatives to provide.

When a person gets no relief from pain through common, routinely available treatments, it makes sense to seek out a center that is specialized in dealing with the most difficult cases of back pain. Because such a center has more options to explore, back surgery sinks to the bottom of a long list. And rightly so. Back surgery should always be a last-ditch effort.

Self-fulfilling prophecies and other ways to increase pain

It is our experience that self-employed individuals are less likely to be disabled from work because of back pain. Perhaps this is because they won't collect benefits, and the businesses that they have struggled their entire lives to build would crumble without them. One may argue that the pain they experience is no different, but rather it is their attitude toward pain that distinguishes them. Or it may be that they are more innovative about getting the job done in alternate ways that don't hurt their backs.

One of the most interesting characteristics of the Texas Back Institute, and why its approach is so effective at relieving back pain, is that it looks at the problems created by disabling back pain through the other end of the telescope.

While the physician is greatly concerned about the individual's pain, the Institute's programs focus on the functions that are affected by pain. Not only does this approach give us a yardstick by which to measure the pain and subsequent improvement, but we've also found that by focusing on activity, people channel their minds and energies into something other than the ol' aching back. This diversion, in turn, tells the brain to think about something else besides the message of pain it is receiving from the nerves. And by getting active, the body begins to produce its own chemical painkillers, endorphins and enkephalins, that can mask the pain.

When a person anticipates waking up in the morning with a backache and doesn't look forward to anything better than lying on the couch and watching television, the expectation of back pain can become a self-fulfilling prophecy. As the person becomes less and less active, joint capsules begin to shrink and muscles atrophy. The more muscles atrophy and weaken, the more susceptible they are to future strain and hence future pain. Over time, if left alone, the downward spiral caused by chronic back pain can suck a person's life right down the drain.

For years, the Texas Back Institute was unique in its emphasis on activity after injury. Unlike other doctors who relied heavily on bed rest, the Texas Back Institute encouraged patients to be active almost immediately. Recently, in 1986, a formal, independent study published in the *New England Journal of Medicine* confirmed the Texas Back Institute's long-standing philosophy of encouraging activity after only two days of bed rest following back injury. The same philosophy of active rehabilitation is now the rule of thumb in the field of sports medicine. Athletes today begin rehabilitation and movement as early as possible after injury — even with the pain of building up an injured knee or arm.

Pain and the self-healing back

Having focused on the many possible causes of back pain, it is important at this point to stress again that the vast majority of back pain — 80 percent — is caused by simple back strain and will cure itself if given enough time and proper exercise. It is known, for example, that within two or three weeks 70 percent of people will get better, and by 12 weeks, 80 percent will feel better.

Remember, the worst part about your first incident of back pain is the fear and anxiety that something really bad and permanent has been done to your back and that you'll need surgery to get rid of the pain. Chances are you are part of the 80 percent mentioned above, and your attack of back pain is merely a signal . . . just pay attention to it.

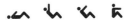

3

Are you a setup for back injury?

ver watch a good western movie? Ever notice that the most successful Indian attacks happened when the Indians waited until dark? Then without making a noise, they would sneak up on the cowboys, who were often bushed from a long day on the range.

Back pain tends to sneak up on us, too. Too often, back pain is a gradual disease that provides few warning signals before it attacks. Just when we think we've gotten away with years of bad posture and bad lifting mechanics, we can be lifting a 12-pack of beer out of the car trunk and get hit with a sensation that has been described by some as being on the business end of a 440-volt cattle prod. We never cease to see the incredulous back owner in our offices mumbling, "Gee, doc, this never happened to me before . . ."

What seemed to be a perfectly pain-free and healthy back ultimately gets strained when you are simply trying to lift a grocery bag. Or digging a golf ball out of heavy rough with a nine iron on the way down the first hole. In other bizarre cases, people have even herniated discs in their spine just by sneezing.

Never mind how it happens; when it does, the resulting back pain can be excruciating. It can extend down into the legs or arms, or freeze a person in a contorted, painful pose. Indeed, the comedy act that portrays the poor victim of back pain in a perverse, frozen, half-bent-over position is not entirely inaccurate. When this happens, it's usually Mother Nature's way of keeping us from doing any further damage to our backs.

The good news in all this is that for most of us, the first incident of back pain won't be serious. Most likely the pain will go away with rest and time. Few people recognize that back pain is a signal that something is wrong. Ignoring that signal is asking for real trouble — the kind that stays with you for life.

The majority of back problems are related to muscle and ligament strain. The Egyptian pharaohs were among the first to complain about back pain, since they did most of their work from their thrones. Similarly, in today's automated world, those with sedentary jobs and lifestyles — who also add inches to their waistlines — make their backs more vulnerable to injury.

How does a big belly affect the back? As the stomach protrudes, it can pull forward on the alignment of the low back, setting it up for injury. Pregnant women often experience back pain in the last months of pregnancy.

Finally, a cholesterol level for your back

Ten years ago, how many people knew what the word *cholesterol* meant? Over the last decade, thanks to the American Heart Association, almost every American knows what cholesterol is, how it affects the heart, and what foods lower the chances of having a heart attack.

Unfortunately, the field of spine care has not enjoyed

the same awareness. But that is changing. If the eighties were the decade of heart awareness, the nineties will be the decade of spine awareness.

Why? Because health care costs are escalating out of control. And a big portion of this health-care bill is from disability, that is, the money that must be paid to people who cannot work because of their injuries. Back problems are by far the leading cause of disability for people 18 to 55 years old. By contrast, arm pain may be troublesome, but it probably will not permanently prevent someone from working. Severe back pain, however, can be crippling.

Also, once a back is injured, it sometimes becomes a matter of damage control. If the injury is severe enough that surgery is required to repair the damage, there will be a long road back through rehabilitation, and the individual may have to adjust his or her activities to prevent a reinjury.

Just as measurement of cholesterol levels has proven to be a ground-breaking tool for assessing our personal risk of future heart attack, there are new ways in the field of spine care to determine a person's individual risk of back injury.

Using a new procedure called computerized isokinetic testing, a spine specialist can measure the strength of a person's back and get a pretty good picture of whether the person has a back injury waiting to happen.

In a sitting position, the person extends backward and then forward. There is no weight to lift. Instead, resistance is produced in direct proportion to the amount of torque created by the person. The stronger a person's back, the more resistance, and the more torque registered on the computer. The all-important numbers produced by this test show how a person's back and abdominal strength compares to the average strength of others of the same body weight who have no back impairment.

Ideally, the extensor muscles in the back would generate at least the same amount of peak torque in foot-pounds as body weight. Equally important, the ratio between the extensor muscles and the abdominal muscles should be at least three to two.

A 180-pound man, for example, should be able to produce at least 180 foot-pounds of torque with his back muscles and at least 120 foot-pounds of torque with his stomach muscles. Anything less would imply that either his extensors or his abdominals, or both, need to be strengthened to avoid future back strain.

How do most people measure up? It varies tremendously. Oil field workers from West Texas who have been tested at the Texas Back Institute have generated monstrous back strength equal to 200 percent of their body weight. Keep in mind, however, that these roustabouts spend 40 hours a week throwing chains and jerking heavy pipe while standing on an oily metal derrick platform.

On the other end of the spectrum, most people who have desk jobs and do little lifting either on the job or in their off hours will fall way short of matching 100 percent of their body weight in measuring torque produced by either back or abdominal muscles.

In a way, these people are at similar risk of back strain as oil field workers. The only difference may be the kind of back injury sustained. It may take a lot of stress or weight to strain the back muscles of a strong oil field worker. For a sedentary person, however, lifting a bag of grass clippings from the lawn mower may be enough to cause an injury.

Also, because of the nature of the job the individual must return to after recovering from a back injury, the oil field worker is more likely to be disabled than the person who performs a desk job.

What is your risk of back injury?

Knowing your risk of back pain is helpful because it can act as a catalyst for change. For some people, finding out that their cholesterol level is at 280 is like discovering they have a bomb ready to go off inside their chest. Suddenly, when faced with the ominous prospect of impending heart attack, diet improves instantaneously and exercise becomes an all-important part of the day.

Aside from isokinetic testing, you can assess your overall risk of back injury by evaluating your daily and recreational activities as well as your overall fitness.

Do you have a high-risk job?

Garbage collectors, nurses, and people whose jobs require them to lift things place continual demand on their backs. The inherent danger in these jobs usually comes from
- not warming up at the beginning of the day
- becoming fatigued at the end of the day
- trying to lift something heavier than normal

Do you have a desk job that requires you to sit most of the day?

Sitting for extended periods of time actually stresses the back. It also does little to strengthen the back. Even walking, bending, and lifting small objects throughout the day acts somewhat as an exercise maintenance program for the back. A sedentary job can set up a back injury when matched with heavy weekend-warrior activity.

Are you overweight by more than 20 percent?

Experts haven't established a concrete connection between obesity and back pain. But many specialists believe having a large stomach tends to pull the spine forward out of alignment, which then sets the stage for back strain.

One thing is for sure: being overweight creates extra stress on your back and probably makes it difficult — if not impossible — to maintain an exercise and fitness program. Here is a brief list of heights and the recommended weight for each. If you exceed this recommended weight by more than 20 percent, clinically speaking, you are obese and should seek out a weight control program.

Height	Women's Weight	Men's Weight
4'11"	106	
5'0	109	116
5'1"	112	119
5'2"	116	122
5'3"	120	125
5'4"	124	128
5'5"	128	131
5'6"	133	136
5'7"	136	142
5'8"	140	147
5'9"	144	152
5'10"	148	158
5'11"		166
6'0"		172
6'1"		178
6'2"		184
6'3"		189
6'4"		195

To determine the percentage above or below ideal body weight

Sample	Man 6'0"	Woman 5'3"
Current body weight:	185	148
minus ideal weight:	− 172	− 120
equals pounds above/below:	13	28
Divide by ideal weight:	13/172 =.07	28/120 =.23
Multiply by 100:	.07 x 100 = 7%	.23x100 =23%
Result:	7% overweight	23% overweight

Do you participate in high-risk sports such as football, downhill skiing, dirt biking, water skiing, weight lifting, racquetball, tennis, or golf?

Some studies note that less than 10 percent of sports injuries involve the spine. There are certain sports that have higher risk, however.

Golf is a prime example. One study notes that touring pros have a 29 percent incidence of acute or chronic low back complaints throughout their careers. In fact, 90 percent of all tour injuries involve the neck or back. Considering that the head of a driver at impact is traveling at speeds of more than 130 miles an hour and that the swing takes only two seconds, imagine the torque placed on the spine to generate a powerful golf shot.

Football is tough on the back just because it's a contact sport. For blockers and linemen, football can present special problems because they are pushing and receiving impact in a hyperextended, or arched back, posture.

Skiing and dirt biking are jackhammer sports. They force the spine to absorb great repetitive shock. And in the case of falls, there is a large chance of traumatic injury to vertebrae, rather than just muscle strain.

Racquetball is probably the most dangerous racket sport. Not to mention that ophthalmologists have dealt with thousands of eye injuries from the sport, the mechanics of the racquetball stroke are murder on the back. When the game is played properly — with the ball kept low and struck just inches off the court floor — the player must coil and then untwist, all the while in a semi-bent posture.

If you answered yes to any of these questions, consider yourself at higher than normal risk for a future back injury. Managing that risk is what the following chapters on exercise are all about.

If you still question the need for worrying about back injury ahead of time, consider the following: research has shown that once you have a back injury, you are four times as likely to have a recurrence. It's unfortunate, but the back indeed has a memory.

Which is why prevention of the first injury is so all-important, and why any type of minor back pain should grab your attention. Back pain is a warning signal. Listen to it. Act on it. Get your back in shape.

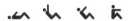

Back care in the nineties: Championing a sports medicine approach

The following scene takes place every day at the Texas Back Institute. Bill, a busy executive, visits the clinic for relief of acute back pain. He is noticeably relieved when the physician tells him he has nothing more serious than a muscle strain, but the following news flash catches him off guard.

"We'll start with some anti-inflammatories and physical therapy to lessen the pain, and then get you into a solid exercise program to strengthen that back," the physician reports. The look on Bill's face says it all. Instant anguish . . . as if someone had punched him in the sore spot in his low back. "You've got to be kidding, Doc!" Bill squirms. "Exercise? My back is killing me. The last thing I want to do right now is exercise."

The sports medicine approach to recovery

Sentencing Bill to what he perceives to be an exercise dungeon would be cruel if it were not that recent research has proven that the best way to treat back pain and other orthopedic problems is not through passive treatments but through active rehabilitation — which includes exercise.

Much of this research has its origins in sports medicine. A decade ago it was common for physicians to immobilize injured arms and legs in traction and plaster casts through long periods of inactivity. Athletes challenged this treatment philosophy, however, by impatiently pushing their doctors to allow them to return to their sports quicker after injury.

This sports medicine approach of active rehabilitation has shown that the former passive treatment of rest and inactivity makes recovery more difficult and in some cases impossible. Muscles atrophy and joint capsules shorten, making movement and returning to activity more painful.

From a physiological standpoint, the overall physical capacity of the cardiovascular and musculoskeletal systems decreases rapidly with their disuse, leading to decreased muscle size, strength, endurance, and work capacity, as well as decreases in an individual's ability to participate in the normal activities of daily living. The end result is that the person becomes even more susceptible to strain and future injury. In short, a continual downward spiral leads to more inactivity and disability.

By forcing the person to return to activity, the muscles and cardiovascular system have less time to atrophy, and the road back to full strength is easier and quicker.

The second benefit of exercise is that it stimulates the body's production of its own natural painkillers, called endorphins and enkephalins. Exercise has been shown to increase the body's secretion of endorphins, which are believed to be responsible for the self-induced euphoria known as "runner's high." Not only do these natural morphines raise a person's threshold for pain, but they enhance mood and combat depression. Just as someone can become dependent on drugs, runners can become dependent on their exercise fix. It's not unusual to see avid runners outside in snow and rain rather than skip their daily exercise fix and spend the day feeling down rather than feeling up.

Without exercise, production of endorphins and other mood enhancers falls off dramatically. Consequently, one must incorporate exercise into the daily routine to enjoy not only the benefits to strength and endurance but also the painkilling effects produced.

Not surprisingly, the role of exercise in the management and prevention of back injuries is steadily increasing. The sports medicine approach is in fact a broad approach that takes into account physiological, psychological, nutritional, biomechanical, pathological and environmental factors.

Exercise is a very general term for a variety of specific activities. Exercise in a rehabilitation setting must be prescribed cautiously because it may either help or hinder efforts to treat a back injury. There are essentially four different general classifications of rehabilitative exercise: *active*, *resistive*, *passive*, and *functional*.

Active exercise

Active exercises are those that can be completed by the patient without assistance. These types of movements are generally less stressful to the patient than other kinds of exercise when performed correctly.

Active exercises require coordinated activity by the muscles and tendons and the neural systems that stimulate these tissues, increasing their functional capacity.

An individual's range of motion, or flexibility, can be assessed by a therapist or exercise physiologist through active exercise. Because pain normally limits active movement, the individual will avoid performing movements that cause pain. Accordingly, by having the individual in control, the risk of additional injury to a damaged area is reduced.

Resistive exercise

Resistive exercises can help the therapist or exercise

physiologist further assess the integrity of the muscles, tendons, and related neural tissues. Resistive exercises also stimulate and stress these muscle tissues better than normal active exercises.

The best example of a resistive exercise is lifting a weight. The nerves, muscles, and tendons must all work in a coordinated fashion to perform the lift, where the weight acts as the resistance to the tissues.

Muscular strength is measured by resistive exercises. By definition, strength is the maximum amount of force that can be developed by a muscle. It takes more strength, for instance, to lift a 100-pound weight than a 50-pound weight. Because muscles in the back act as guy wires, holding bony vertebrae in place under stress, increasing muscular strength can help stabilize a joint that moves too much.

Also, if the back and stomach muscles become stronger, the amount of weight that the spine has to support is decreased. This is one of the most important benefits of a back rehabilitation program.

Muscular endurance is often viewed as being the same as muscular strength. But muscular endurance, as compared to muscular strength, is not a measure of how much strength or force a muscle can generate or how much weight can be lifted by a muscle. Instead, muscular endurance is more a measure of how long a muscle can continue to work at less-than-maximum effort.

For example, it takes more endurance to lift a 50-pound weight 30 times than it does to lift the same weight 15 times. In a back rehabilitation program, by increasing an individual's level of muscular endurance, the individual will be able to do more work before his or her muscles fatigue. Fatigue, as you remember from earlier chapters, is a prime culprit in many back injuries.

Cardiovascular endurance exercises are a combination of active and resistive exercises. They increase the volume of blood delivered to the exercising tissues. This blood carries oxygen and other vital components required to repair damaged tissues. In addition, the blood also transports many energy-rich nutritional components to both injured and uninjured tissues, which enables the tissues to exercise or function longer and more efficiently.

In addition, this increased delivery of blood also increases tissue temperature, which may allow tissues to stretch, move, and function more effectively with less dysfunction, pain, and related symptoms. Finally, cardiovascular exercise also helps the exercising muscles to flush out lactic acid, a metabolic by-product that tends to accumulate in the muscles.

Lactic acid acts as nature's chemical circuit breaker. It is this chemical that causes the muscle to shut down, or fatigue, the harder it is worked. The stronger and more conditioned the muscle, however, the less lactic acid build-up. Consequently, an active cardiovascular system helps muscle tissues become stronger and more resistant to fatigue.

Passive exercise

Passive exercises are those that are performed by a device, by a therapist, or by the patient without contracting the muscle. Generally, passive exercises are used to assess the function of bones, joints, ligaments, and other tissues. In a rehabilitative setting, they are usually used to assess or increase flexibility.

An example of a passive exercise is the hamstring stretch performed with a rope. A rope is placed around the bottom of the foot, with the ends in each hand. The foot and leg are lifted passively by employing the strength of the muscles of the upper body to pull on the rope. The hamstring muscle is stretched passively in this fashion, without having to lift the leg by using the musculature of the leg. Because the potential to increase the level of pain or worsen an injury is greater than with other types of exercise, care should be used when performing passive exercises on an injured area.

Sometimes pain arises when tight tissues surrounding a joint restrict or modify its normal movement. Pain may also occur from a muscle spasm, which may be caused by decreased blood supply to an area. Flexibility exercises stretch and lengthen tight muscles, tendons, and ligaments, enabling nearby joints to move more freely and correctly. In both cases, stretching of tight muscles can help control pain as well as treat the underlying cause.

Functional exercise

Functional exercises are those activities or movements that simulate work or daily activities. For a warehouse worker, for example, functional exercises could include lifting differently shaped boxes with varying weights inside. Functional exercises help an injured person to return to work by strengthening specifically those muscle groups that will be needed back on the job.

Back pain often occurs because the person was out of shape beforehand. As a result of back injury, muscles may atrophy, making the recovery process more difficult. The earlier exercise can be introduced into the individual's treatment program, the faster and easier recovery will be. More important, exercise is proven by medical research to show lasting benefit. By strengthening weak muscles, the individual's back becomes injury resistant rather than injury prone.

PART II

Stacking the Odds
in Your Favor

5

Exercises you can do at home to get your back in shape

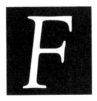or those interested in preventing back pain, or those with sporadic back pain, maintaining a back exercise program is the best way to prevent future back pain attacks. The goals of a back exercise program are to

- strengthen extensor muscles, the main lifters in the back
- strengthen the abdominal muscles that support and align the spine
- strengthen the stabilizer muscles of the body trunk
- strengthen the leg muscles that share lifting duty with the back
- improve flexibility

Equipment you'll need to buy

Nothing.

An effective home exercise program doesn't require thousands of dollars' worth of sophisticated training apparatus.

Most people possess all of the required equipment for a back exercise program right in their own homes.

Here's what you'll really need: motivation and determination. Sure, it's easy to get motivated to start an exercise program to get rid of annoying back pain attacks. But staying with it? That takes determination.

Most people diet to reach a target weight, for instance. And many people through sheer willpower reach their target. Unfortunately, they often put the weight right back on because they have failed at behavior modification. In other words, they have not incorporated a new eating style into their lives. When they stop dieting, over-eating resumes and the fat goes right back on.

Similarly, a back exercise program is not something you do for a while, then put up on the shelf. As any bodybuilder will testify, slacking off on workouts lets muscles atrophy. Simply put, if you don't use 'em, you lose 'em. The best advice is to incorporate the home exercise program into your daily activities — just like brushing your teeth. Go through your exercises either in the morning or evening, or at lunchtime. Whatever works for you. Just be consistent. That way, it will be harder to get out of the habit.

Flexibility exercises

It is important that you not only strengthen your back and stomach muscles, but also improve flexibility. Golf, for example, doesn't require much back strength but it does require exceptional flexibility. *Golf Digest* notes that 75 percent of all pro golf injuries occur in the spine. Of those, half occur in the low back, where the turn, slide, twist, and tilt of the golf swing wreak havoc. And this is among professionals with typically smooth, grooved swings. Amateur golfers with jerky swings and unconditioned backs — beware.

Warm-up exercises

Each exercise session should start off with a general

warm-up that includes light stretching to warm and lengthen tight musculoskeletal structures such as muscles, tendons, and ligaments, as well as lubricate joints. In addition, a gradual warm-up is required to slowly increase the work performed by the cardiovascular system.

The major muscle groups of the body — back, chest, shoulders, arms, trunk, and legs — should be stretched in the warm-up. The individual muscles should be slowly stretched to a point of very mild muscular tension, held for a count of 10 to 30 seconds while you breathe normally, and then the muscles should be completely relaxed before the next repetition.

Each stretch should be repeated five times per muscle group. When possible, alternate stretches from one side of the body to the other, right to left, before repeating.

It's important that you don't feel pain from any stretching exercise. The sensation should be like a gradual stretching of the muscle. If a stretch causes a sharp or stabbing pain, try the stretch in a slower fashion or don't stretch the muscle as far. If the stretch increases pain, tingling or numbness in any area, stop. You should probably visit your doctor.

Stretches should be done while lying on the back when forward flexing of the trunk is required. This helps reduce intravertebral disc pressures, which are increased when performing movements in a standing or sitting forward-flexed position.

After the light stretching routine has been completed, the cardiovascular warm-up and conditioning phase may be started. This phase could consist of a slow walk that progresses to a brisk walk. After about five minutes your heart rate should be at least 100 beats a minute. A light perspiration indicates that the body has been sufficiently warmed and is ready for the next stretching phase.

Again, these stretches should be taken to a point of mild tension, where the stretch starts, and then held for 10 to 30 seconds and repeated five times each. Alternate when possible from right to left sides of the body. The muscles may relax somewhat over the course of the stretch. If this occurs, the muscles may be stretched further as long as the above guidelines are adhered to. Remember that mild tension, not pain, is the goal of the stretching routine.

Cardiovascular exercise

After the completion of the stretching phase, emphasis should be on enhancing the efficiency of the heart and lungs as together they deliver much-needed energy and oxygen to the exercising muscles. A light jog or run can accomplish this, or even a walk. Walking uses the large muscle groups of the lower extremities as well as the buttocks and low back muscles to stabilize the spine and upper body. Walking is also easy for most people recovering from a simple back muscle strain.

Duration is the first goal of this type of cardiovascular conditioning program. The ideal back program consists of daily aerobic activity. This might mean getting started with a minimum of a five-minute walk, progressing over the course of four weeks to walks of 20 minutes.

If you prefer to jog or run, remember that the objective of this phase is duration, not intensity. Instead of wind sprints, try to maintain a run at a slower pace for a longer period of time. You may want to invest in a good pair of running or aerobic shoes. Athletic shoe design has progressed dramatically over the last decade. Well-designed shoes provide cushioning and shock absorption when running and jumping, which lessens stress on the knees and the back. Not to mention, your feet will love you for it.

The ultimate goal of this exercise phase is to raise your heart rate to a plateau. For the out-of-shape person, this plateau, or exercise value, might be 60 percent of his or her maximum heart rate. The exercise value for the in-shape person, conversely, might be 85 percent. To determine your exact training zone, which takes into account a variety of factors including age, resting heart rate and current aerobic condition, use the table below. (For individuals taking certain medications, this method of calculating heart rate is not valid and can be dangerous. Consult your doctor or therapist before starting any program.)

How to determine your heart rate range

	Sample 1	Sample 2
Starting point:	220	220
Deduct your age:	– 40	– 20
Subtotal:	180	200
Deduct your resting heart rate:	– 70	– 60
Subtotal:	110	140
Multiply by your exercise value:	x .60	x .85
Subtotal:	66	119
Add back in your resting heart rate:	+ 70	+ 60
Target heart rate:	**136**	**179**
Training zone (±10 beats):	**126 to 146**	**169 to 189**

How to check your heart rate

There are several ways to check your pulse. The measurement of the pulse at the carotid artery at the neck should be avoided if possible, because pressure on this artery slows the heart rate. The pulse should ideally be felt with the index finger and the third finger.

To measure the pulse, count the number of pulsations felt at the wrist in 10 seconds and multiply this number by six to give the number of times that the heart beats in one minute. Remember that it takes at least five minutes at a steady walking pace for the heart rate to plateau.

Measuring of heart rates is not always completely successful for some people because of their inability to find their pulse and because of variations in predicting maximum heart rate. If you find it difficult to check your pulse, try the "talk test."

While walking, an individual should not be short of

breath. If the person cannot say five or six words without taking a deep breath, then the intensity of aerobic exercise is too great and should be decreased until the person can carry on a conversation.

An additional benefit from maintaining the heart at this active plateau rate is that the body may begin to release endorphins, chemicals resembling morphine which can block or mask the sensation of pain. Endorphins are usually not released into the blood stream in any great volume until exercise intensity is maintained above 80 percent of the individual's maximum heart rate.

An alternative to walking or running

If walking or running is not feasible, or perhaps not to your liking, a stationary bicycle or regular bicycle may also be used for the cardiovascular conditioning phase. Again, the principle is to emphasize duration of the exercise, not intensity. The main difference in cycling as compared to walking or running is that much of the individual's body weight is supported by the bike. As a result, cycling may seem easier than walking for some individuals — especially those with back pain. But because cycling doesn't work out the back muscles as well as walking or running, it is the second choice for a home exercise program.

Additionally, if a person has a bulging or ruptured disc, sitting on a bike can increase intravertebral disc pressure. This pressure can present a problem when the body is flexed forward, as would be the case on a bike with the classic racing handlebars. For the person with a bulging or ruptured disc, an upright posture would be better to reduce disc pressures.

Cool down

After completion of the cardiovascular conditioning phase, allow yourself to cool down to prevent blood from pooling in the legs, which could cause a variety of cardiovascular symptoms such as lightheadedness or dizziness. The cool-down should last a minimum of three minutes, depending on the intensity and duration of the exercise session and your own physical condition. A longer cool-down may be needed to help you recover if your cardiovascular workout was especially intense or if you are out of shape. The cool-down is complete when the heart rate has returned to below 100 beats a minute.

Exercises for the back: Isometric versus dynamic

Generally speaking, any exercise intended to increase strength should be performed slowly and methodically to maximize physical gains while decreasing the potential for an injury from the exercise. This means no jerking.

Exercises can be either isometric, in which a specified position is held for a certain length of time, or dynamic, in which a body part is continually moved in a slow, controlled fashion. During both types of strengthening exercises you should concentrate on proper breathing technique, taking slow, deep breaths from the diaphragm. Ideally, you should exhale as you lift a weight or limb and inhale as you lower it. *Avoid holding your breath*.

When incorporating a new exercise into your routine, it's a good idea to do only 10 repetitions to test the body's tolerance to the specific exercise. Repetitions should be increased with the same weight until the individual can complete 40 consecutive repetitions using correct form and technique. When this becomes easy, increase the weight or resistance, but make sure you can do at least 10 repetitions at the new level. Otherwise don't add as much weight or resistance.

Muscles tend to stay in a somewhat shortened position after doing strengthening exercises. In the out-of-shape person, this may cause muscle cramping or spasms. As a precaution against cramps, you may want to repeat some of the warm-up stretches to lengthen the muscles after a workout.

Single knee to chest —
Lying on back, lift one
knee to chest. Hold for 10
seconds with your arms
as shown. Repeat with
other leg.

 You may find this
exercise difficult after a
back pain attack. If so,
move slowly and work up
to the finish positions
shown.

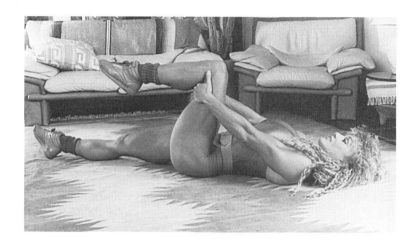

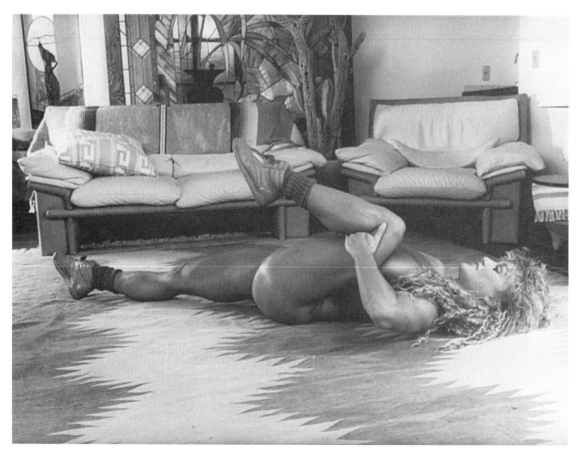

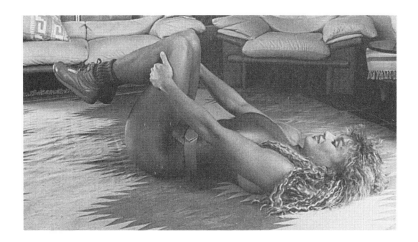

Double knee to chest —
Lying on back, lift one
knee and then the other
to chest. Keep knees
together. Hold for 10
seconds. Lower one leg,
then the other.

Remember to keep
low back in contact with
the floor. Try to lift head
and touch forehead to
knees.

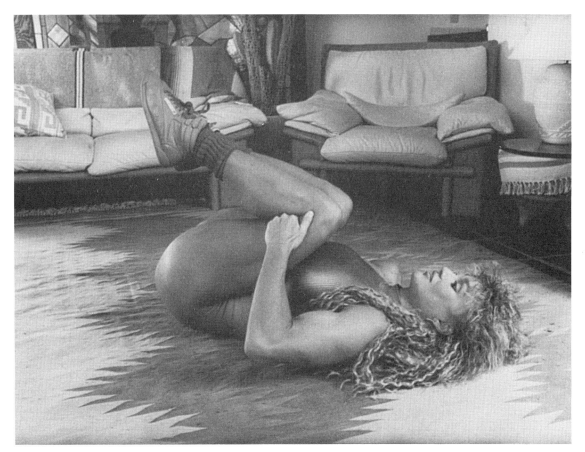

Piriformis stretch — Lie on back with one leg extended. Position other leg with knee bent and crossed over extended leg. Grasp behind bent knee and pull up and across toward opposite shoulder. Hold for 10 seconds.

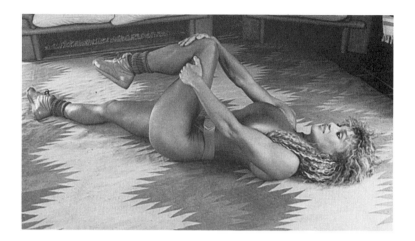

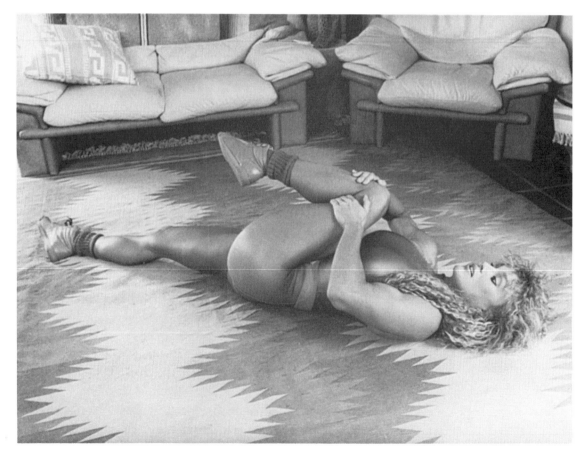

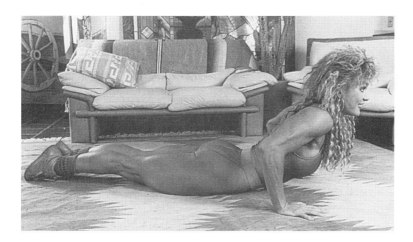

Press-up — Lie on stomach and use arms to slowly raise shoulders. Keeping hips in contact with floor, straighten arms as much as you are able. The aim is to stretch muscles to increase their flexibility. This may be difficult for those people with weak arms, but stick with it.

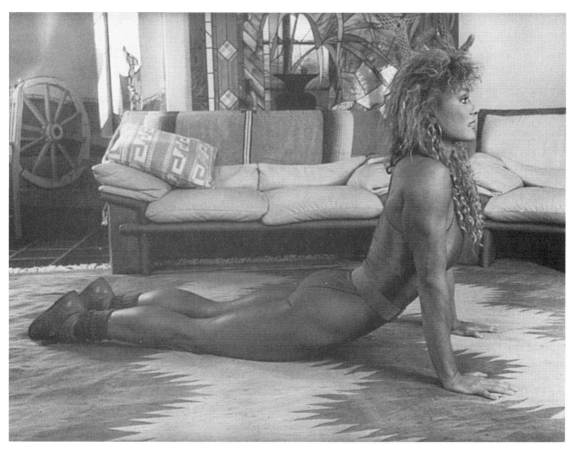

Hip flexor stretch —
Place left knee on towel
and support body weight
by placing hands on right
thigh. Keep back straight.
Slide hips forward until
you feel a slight stretch
on upper left thigh. Hold
for 10 seconds. Repeat
with other leg.

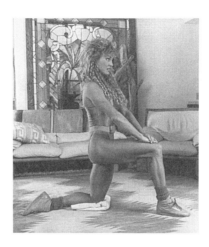

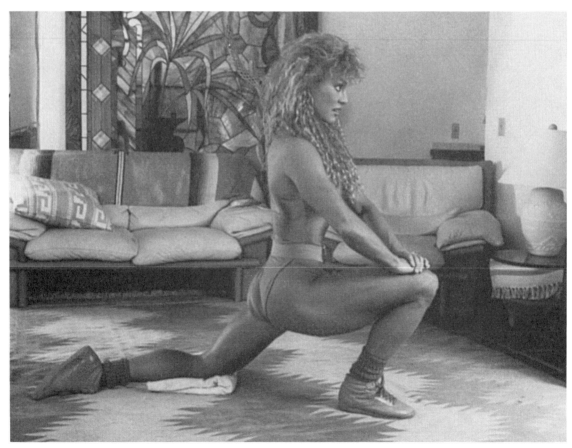

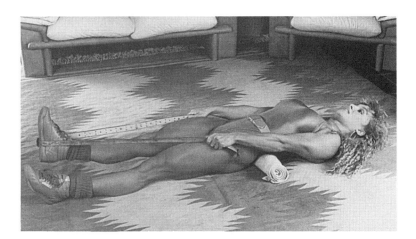

Hamstring stretch — Lie on back with rolled-up towel under curve of back. Keep both legs extended. Place rope or belt around heel of right leg. With knee straight, slowly lift right leg with rope toward chest. Hold for 10 seconds. Repeat with left leg.

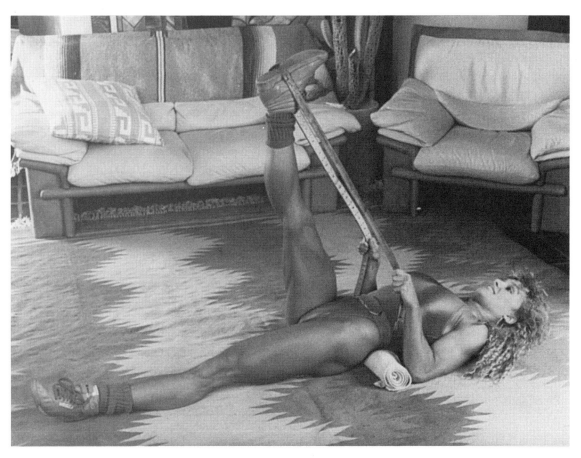

Lumbar rotation — Lie on back with knees bent, heels next to buttocks, shoulders flat, and arms extended. Slowly allow knees to drop toward the floor on one side. Repeat toward other side. Keep shoulders flat throughout the movement. It's okay if your knees at first don't reach the floor.

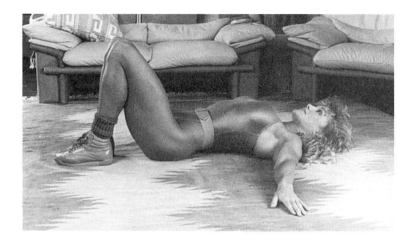

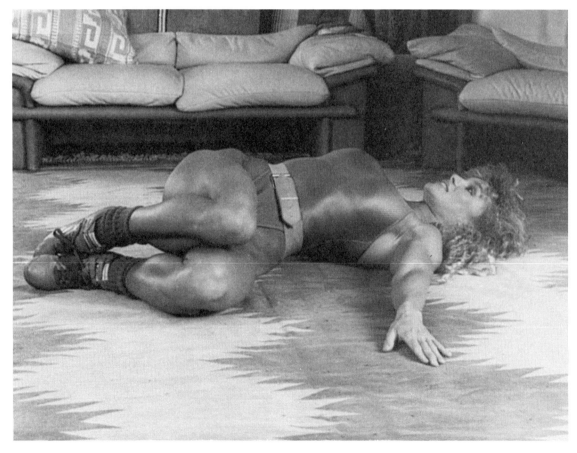

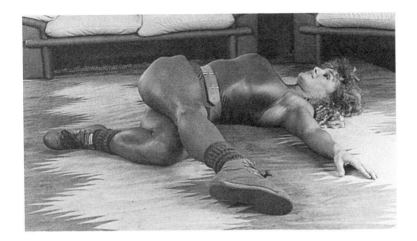

Advanced lumbar rotation — Starting from the finish position on previous exercise, extend top leg out and slowly move arms in the opposite direction of extended leg.

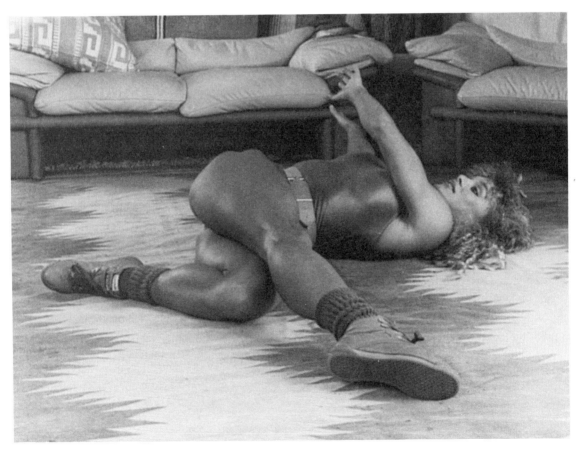

Bridging exercise — Lie on back with heels next to buttocks. Slowly lift buttocks and low back off the floor until thighs and back are in a straight line. Hold for 10 seconds and remember to breathe.

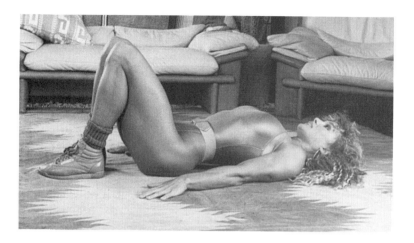

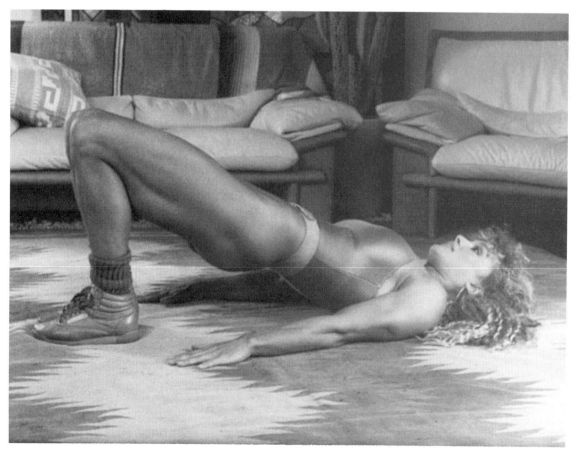

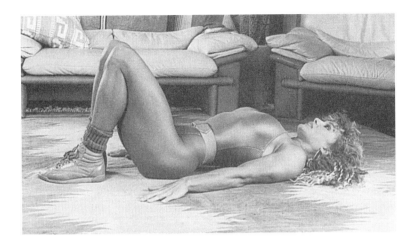

Advanced bridge —
Lie on back with knees
bent and heels next to
buttocks. Lift buttocks
off floor until thighs are
in line with back and
extend the left leg at the
knee. Hold for 10 seconds.
Repeat with other leg and
remember to breathe.

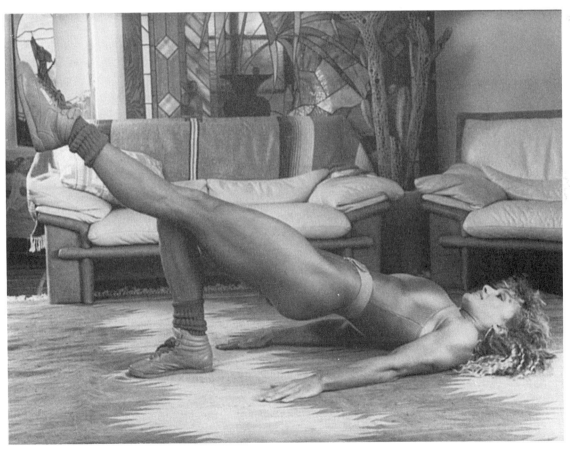

Partial curl — Lie on back with knees bent and heels next to buttocks. Extend hands between thighs. Slowly curl upper torso until shoulder blades leave floor. Hold for 10 seconds. Exhale as you rise.

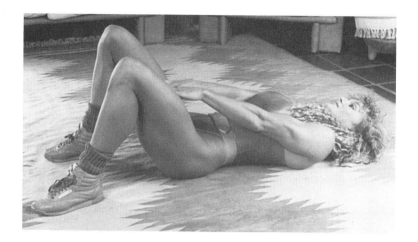

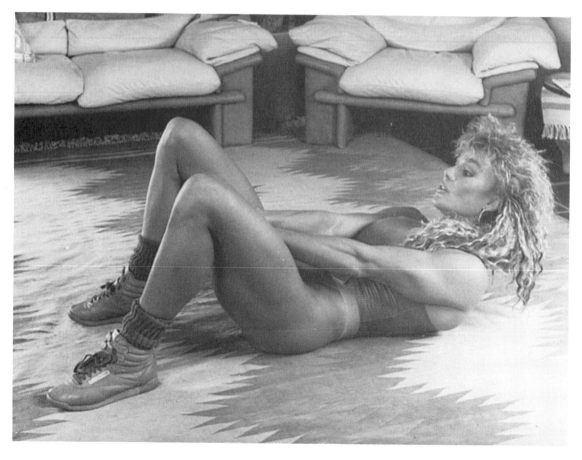

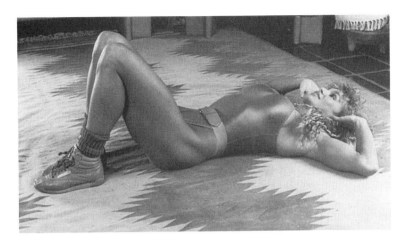

Advanced curl — Lie on back with knees bent, heels next to buttocks, and fingers lightly touching ears. Slowly curl upper torso until shoulders leave the floor. Hold for 10 seconds. Exhale as you rise.

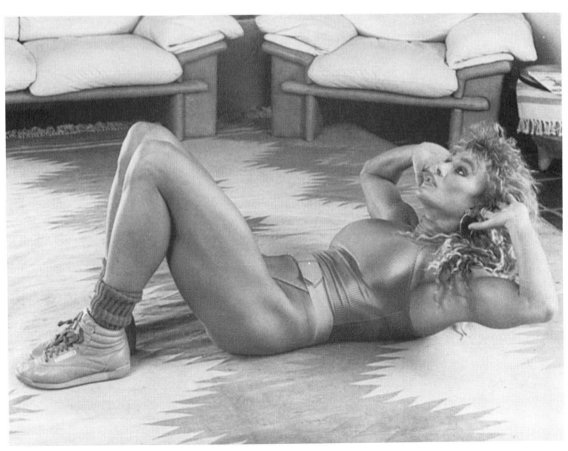

Rotational curl — This exercise works the oblique abdominals. Lie on back with knees bent and heels next to buttocks. Fold arms across chest. Slowly curl right shoulder off floor toward the left knee until left shoulder leaves floor. Hold for 10 seconds, breathing deeply.

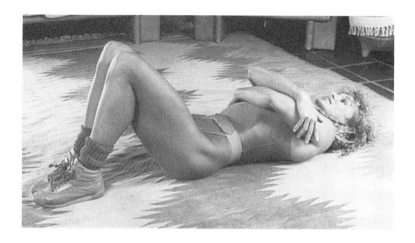

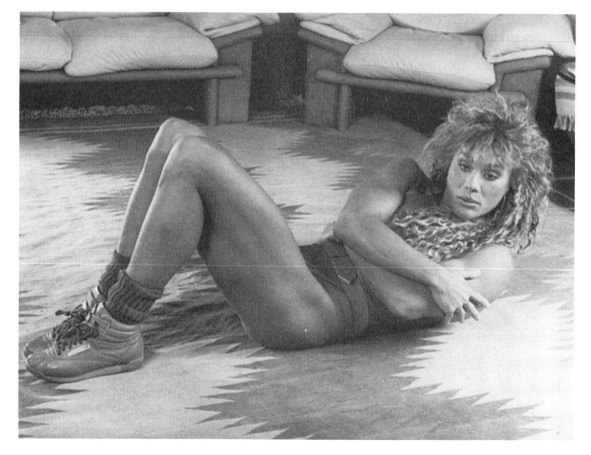

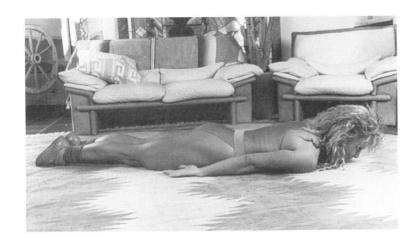

Active spinal extension —
Lie on stomach face
down, arms to side.
Exhale and slowly lift
upper torso off floor.
Hold for 10 seconds.
Remember to breathe.

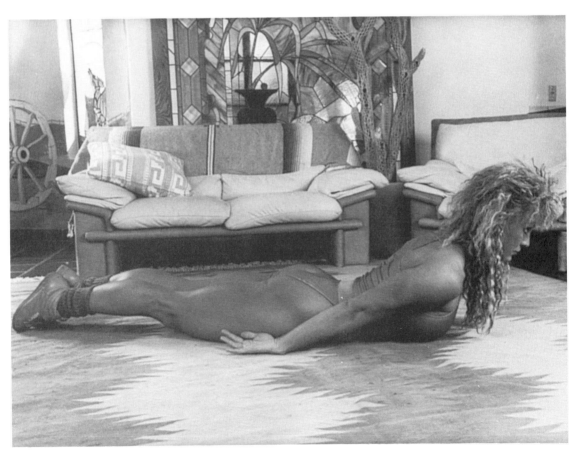

Intermediate spinal extension — Lie face down on stomach with elbows bent and fingers lightly touching ears. Exhale as upper body is lifted off the floor. Hold for 10 seconds. Remember to breathe.

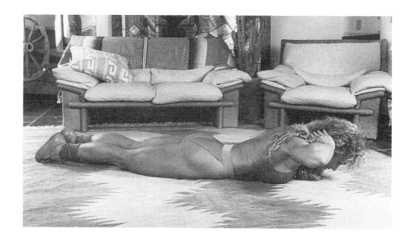

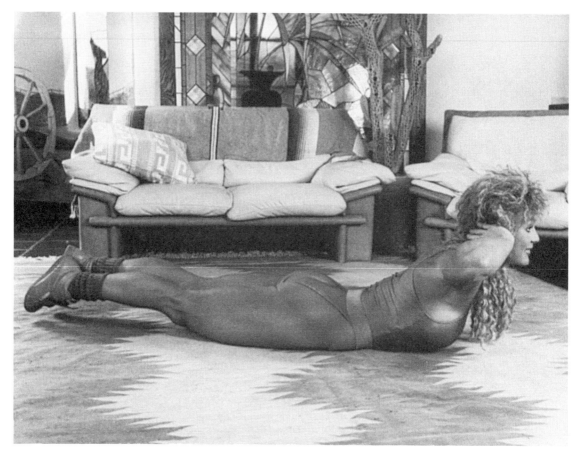

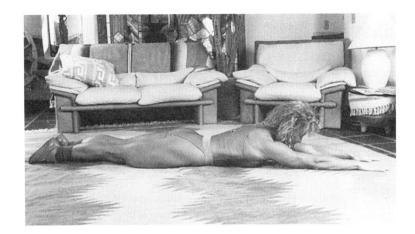

Advanced spinal extension — Lie face down on stomach with arms extended on floor in front of body. Exhale as body is lifted off floor. Hold for 10 seconds. Remember to breathe.

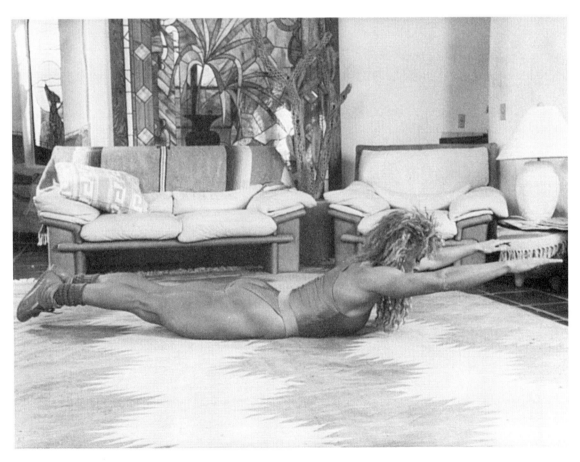

Quadriplex exercises —
(1) Extend right arm.
(2) Extend left leg.
(3) Extend both right arm
and left leg simultaneously.

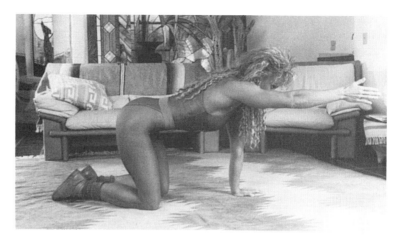

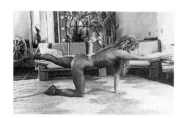

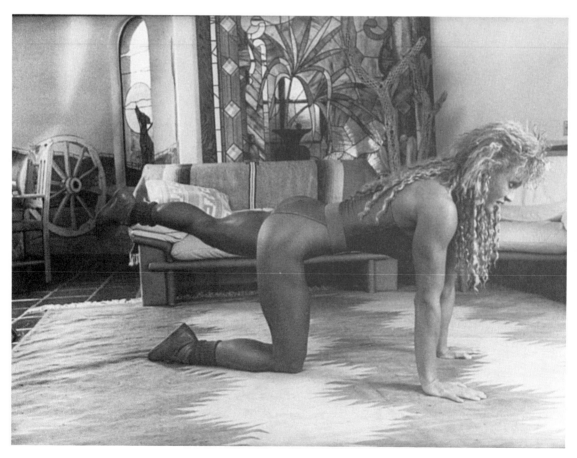

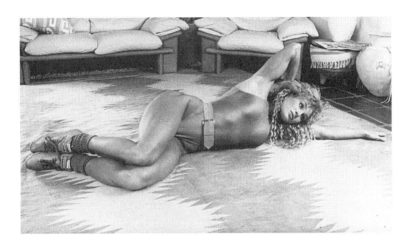

Lateral curl — Lie on left side with knees bent and hips flexed. Slowly lift upper torso up until left shoulder leaves floor. Hold for 10 seconds. Repeat on other side.

This exercise can be tough at first. Still, you are accomplishing something just by feeling your side muscles flex.

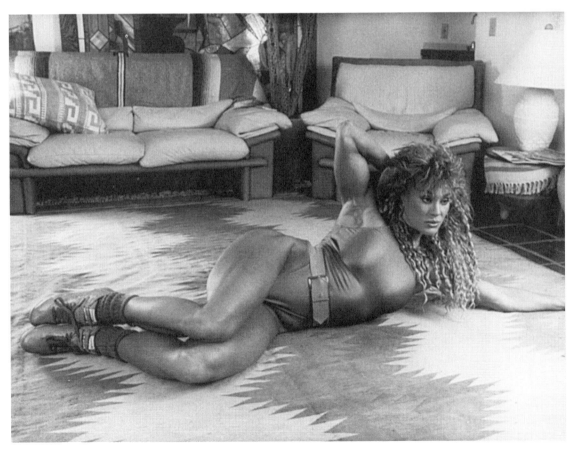

Advanced seated extension — Sit upright with back straight and feet slightly wider than shoulder width apart. Lean slightly forward while keeping the back straight. Hold for 10 seconds. Remember to breathe.

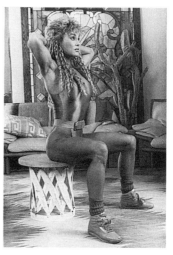

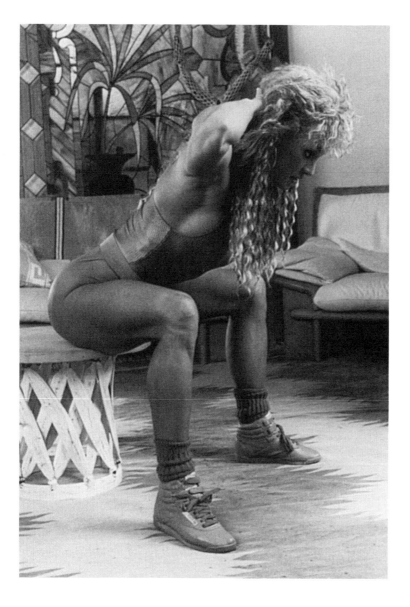

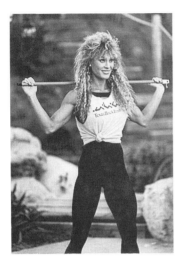

Standing back rotation — Standing straight with back straight and knees slightly bent, place a broomstick over shoulders. Slowly rotate upper torso to left while keeping back straight. Hold for 10 seconds. Repeat to other side and remember to breathe.

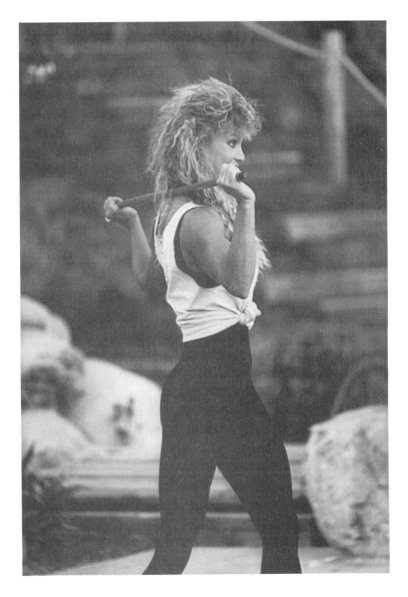

Partial squat — Stand straight with feet shoulder width apart and knees slightly bent. With weight balanced on balls of feet, slowly drop buttocks toward ground while keeping the back straight. Hold for 10 seconds and remember to breathe.

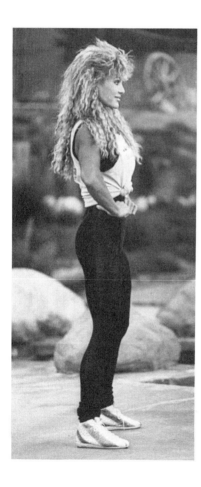 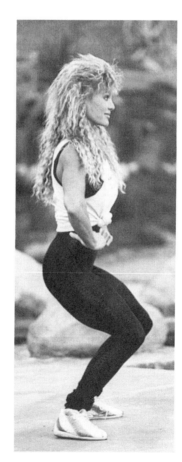

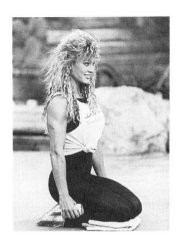

Advanced kneeling extension — With back straight, tighten abdominals. Holding a can of soda or soup in each hand for weight, extend hands out in front to shoulder height. Slowly lean slightly forward, keeping the back straight. Hold for 10 seconds, and remember to breathe. As you are able, you may want to add weight by using two small dumbbells instead of cans.

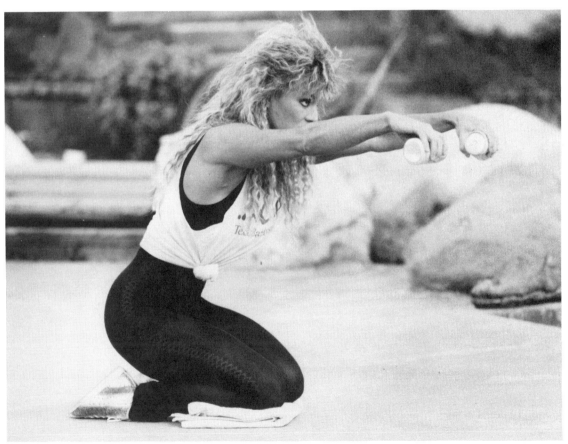

Neck exercise — Top left: Gently press head against hand for 10 seconds. Repeat with other hand. Top right: Rotate head to right, then left, while keeping chin back. Bottom: With chin in, move ear toward shoulder and hold for 10 seconds.

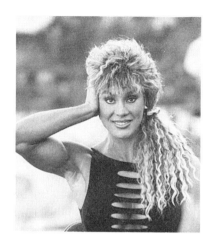

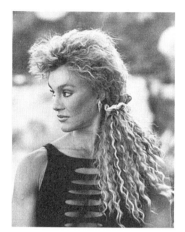

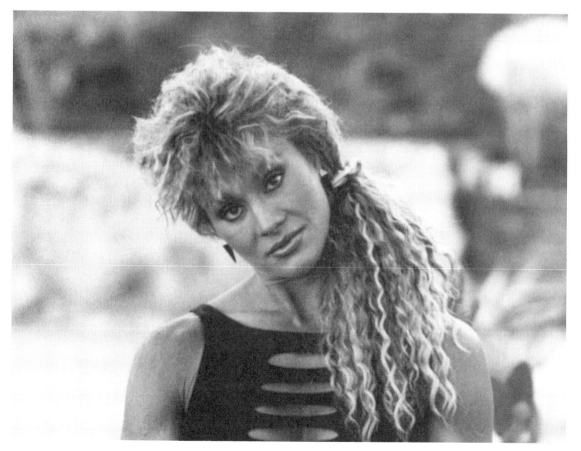

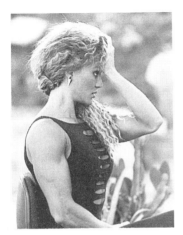

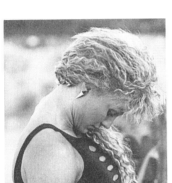

Neck exercise — Top left: With head upright and chin in, lightly press head into hand. Bottom left: Slowly curl chin toward chest. Bottom right: With chin in and mouth closed, slowly extend head backward. Stop exercise if dizziness or lightheadedness occurs. Hold for 10 seconds.

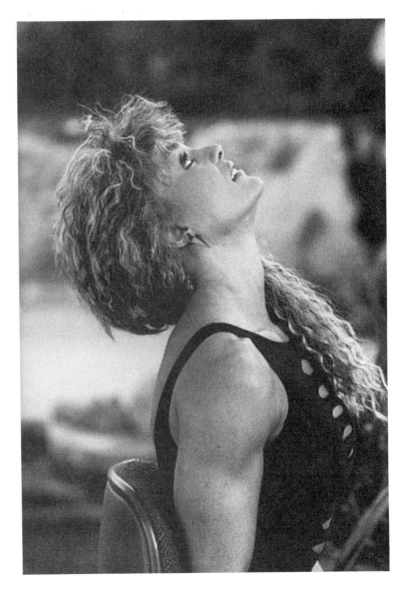

The exercises shown in this chapter can help to manage back pain and decrease future risk of back injury. Select those exercises that you think work best for you, and incorporate them into your daily routine. Some people find that they enjoy doing their back exercises while watching television. Others use their exercise program to get their day off to an active start. Do whatever feels best to you. And keep at it.

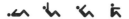

6

Exercises for your gym workout

By now, you know how important it is to strengthen the extensor muscles in the back. Unlike our thigh muscles, which get a daily workout just by supporting the full weight of our bodies as we walk, climb stairs, and run, the back extensor muscles often live a sheltered life. Worse, while thigh muscles are long, powerful muscle strands, the back's extensor muscles resemble a series of short rubber bands that pass from one vertebra to another. It takes a lot of teamwork to get all these muscles working together to get us to stand erect or lift something heavy. And because they are shorter than the long thigh muscles, the extensors are much more prone to spasm and injury.

If you're a young guy interested in working out a little to impress your date, chances are your extensor muscles are the wimpiest muscles you have. This is ironic since they have the toughest real-life demands placed on them.

Visit any gym and you'll notice that guys spend most

of their time around the bench press developing big pectorals and hard biceps — which makes sense because those are the muscles that are most impressive. Women similarly focus on aerobics to control overall weight and use weights to tone their legs, arms, and chest.

But how often do you see anyone using the back extension machine? It's easy to spot in the gym. It's the one with the dust on the seat.

Granted, who gets turned on at the sight of a big muscular back? Understandably, big pectorals may be more sexy. But if you're using a gym to build up, don't forget to invest a little time building up the extensors that do most of the dirty work of lifting and carrying all day long.

At some point you may want to strengthen to a level beyond what is possible through a home program. Or you may find that with distractions or diversions at home, it's easier to keep on your exercise program by joining a gym and making it part of your daily routine, either first thing in the morning, at lunch, or after work in the evening.

Others join gyms or health clubs because they help them stay motivated. Many people find that working out at a gym maintains their motivation because they see all the other people working out. All those healthy positive attitudes rub off on each other. If you find your home program boring, a health club or gym can provide both motivation and virtually limitless variety in exercises.

A health club or gym can also enable you to improve muscle strength dramatically, much more than you could at home without weights or machines. There are many different types of exercise machines, which allow you to develop specific muscle groups to a strength level that would not normally be possible through a home program.

In a home program, the resistance in specific exercises is usually limited to the weight of the body segment that is being lifted. In a fitness facility, however, exercise machines can enable you to ratchet up gradually the resistance placed on a muscle group. By forcing the muscle to lift heavier weight, the muscle becomes stronger.

Some general medical concerns

Some individuals experience problems related to stenosis or narrowing of the spinal canal. Many times, extension exercises or side bending can cause radicular pain, that is, pain that radiates into a leg or arm because nerve roots are compressed or pinched by the vertebrae in this posture. Many exercises can aggravate this condition, but those like the rowing machine, stair-climbing exercises, and treadmill walking or running with excessive grade are especially bad unless the participant limits extension during the activity. In other words, avoid bending backward.

Likewise, individuals with a spondylolisthesis should also avoid extension exercises beyond the neutral position. The neutral position is the normal position of the spine in standing. In neutral, the spine is straight up, not leaning forward nor leaning backward. In spondylolisthesis, a segment or segments of the spine have moved forward on the segments below them. Extension exercises in which you lean backward tend to place more forward forces on the already displaced segments, causing pain and other symptoms and potentially worsening the condition.

Rotation is another movement that can cause pain after an injury to the low back. Furthermore, any movement or exercise activity that requires pelvic rotation will transfer the rotational forces to the low back through the sacrum, oftentimes creating pain and related symptoms. Exercises that have inherent rotational components should be used cautiously.

Jogging and running warrant special attention as exercise activities for the back-injured patient. Jogging and running can be bad for the back because of the impact placed on each segment of the spine as body weight returns to the ground after each stride. Again, a good pair of running shoes, along with improving running form, can help reduce some of these impact forces.

In the worst case, impact forces from running can be as much as four times the person's body weight with each stride. Imagine the long- or even short-term effects of this kind of impact on the spine as well as the lower extremities and joints. Jogging, a slower version of running, creates many more up-and-down forces than does running. Good runners tend to propel the body more forward than up and down. This, theoretically, decreases the impact on the spine. Running may therefore be a better choice than jogging, provided the rotational forces from running are tolerated.

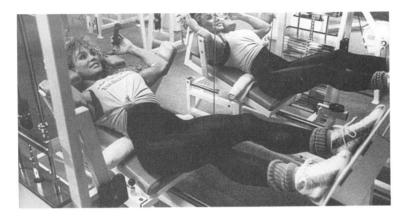

Leg press — Lie on back with a small towel rolled under low back. Place feet shoulder width apart and adjust the seat position until knees do not exceed a 90-degree bend. Slowly press body backward by extending knees and hips. Do not lock knees.

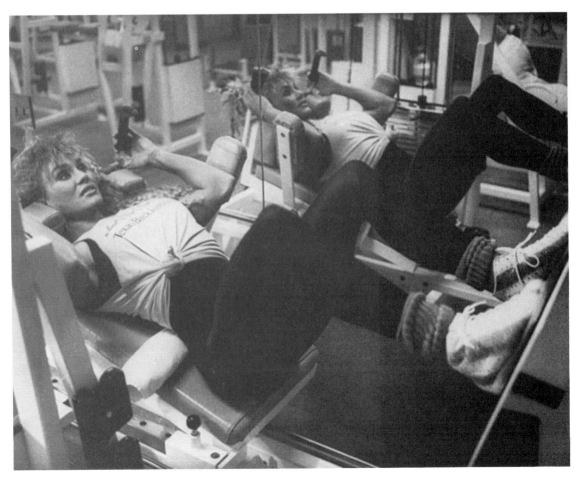

Leg curl — Lie on bench with knees off the edge of the pad. Grasp handles and slowly curl heels toward buttocks, then return to starting position. Do not arch back during the exercise and remember to breathe.

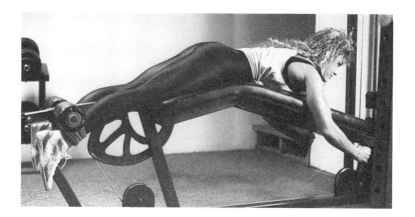

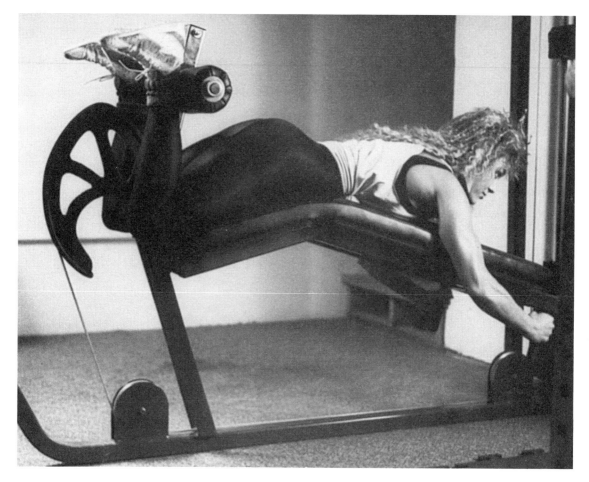

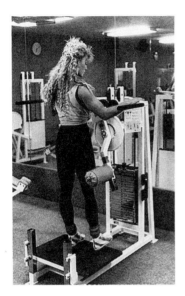

Hip abduction — Standing straight, rest weight on leg. Slowly press outer thigh into pad and raise leg, maintaining upright position of back. Repeat with other leg. Remember to breathe.

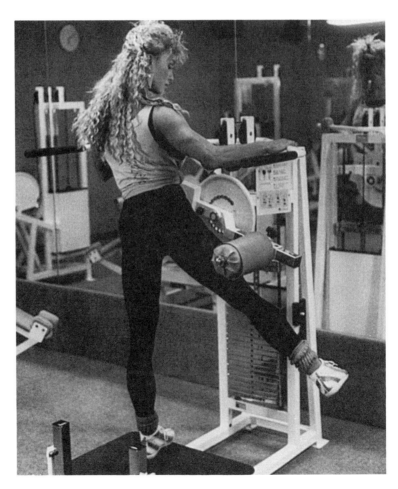

ONE EXERCISE NOT TO DO — Generally, you should avoid doing standing squats with a weighted bar across the neck and shoulders, mainly because there are other ways to work the leg muscles without placing the weight load on the neck. Worse, most beginners do standing squats with an arched or hunched-over spine, which places the back at extreme risk of injury. Cory demonstrates on this page the most common mistakes, and on the next page the correct squat form. Better still, stay away from this exercise altogether.

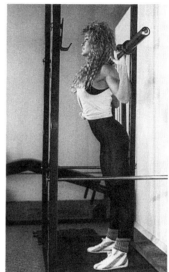

Above, wrong: Back is arched.

Below and left, wrong: Knees and toes are pointed in and the back is rounded forward.

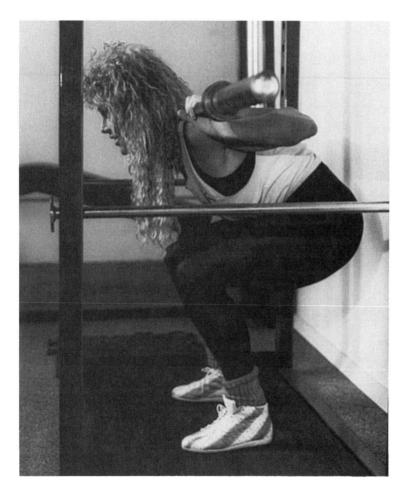

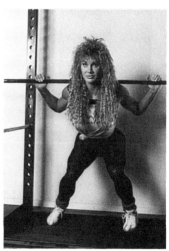

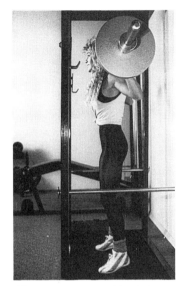

This page shows the correct form for squats. The back is straight, not arched or hunched forward, which allows the weight to be balanced over the middle of the body. Cory looks straight ahead, rather than down at the floor, which also keeps the bar from getting too far forward. For better balance, stand with heels on a small weight or riser.

     The following page shows a better way to exercise the legs with decreased risk to the back.

Above, correct: Back is straight.

Below and right, correct: Knees and toes are pointed out, which provides better balance.

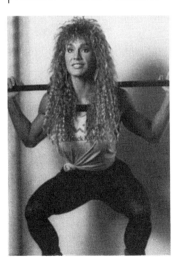

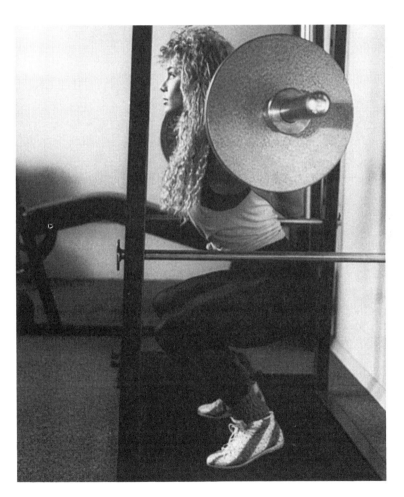

Abdominal exercise — Sit upright with back straight. Tighten abdominals. Fold arms across waist. Slowly flex forward by contracting lower abdominals. Stop forward motion at about a 30-degree angle. Discontinue exercise if pressure is felt in low back. Always follow this exercise with an extension exercise.

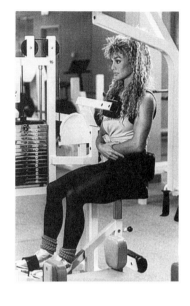

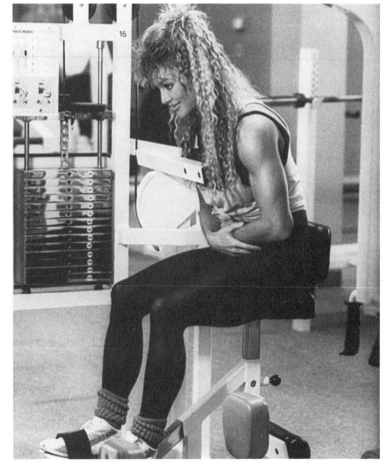

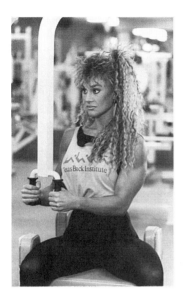

Oblique exercise — Sit upright with buttocks back. Press thighs against pressure pads and slowly rotate upper torso using oblique abdominal muscles, not shoulders or arms. Repeat toward other side. Remember to breathe.

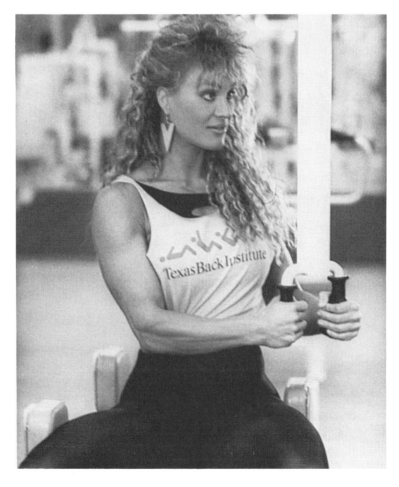

Calf raise — Sit upright with back straight and pressure pad at mid-thigh. Slowly press thighs upward into pressure pad and then return to starting position.

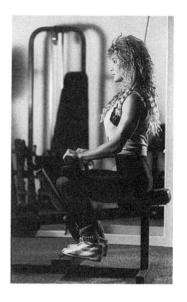

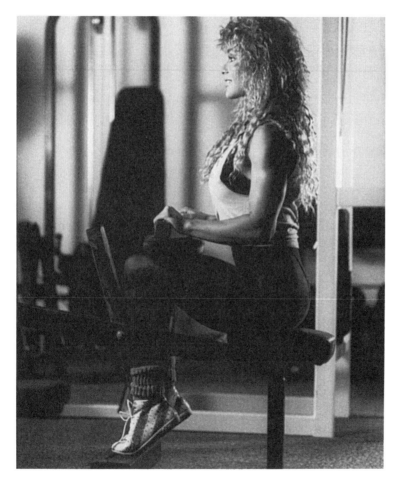

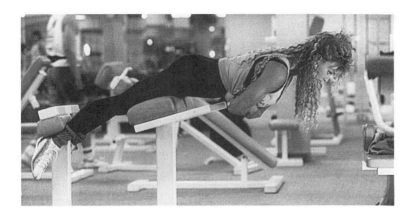

Back extension — Start with back straight and hands folded across chest. Slowly lower upper body and then return to starting position. Hold for five seconds at starting position and repeat. Do not arch back.

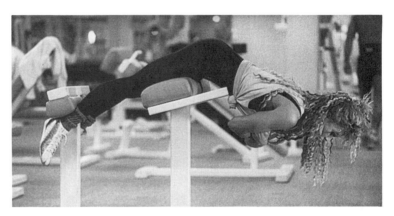

(<u>Note</u>: This exercise can be done on a machine that allows for variable weight and resistance, or on a simple Roman chair, as shown here. On a Roman chair, resistance can be increased by moving hands from across chest to behind head, as shown at right.)

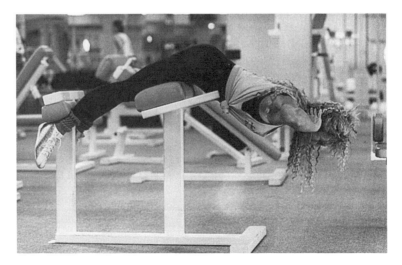

Lat pull-down — Start with back straight, not arched. Tighten abdominals and lean slightly forward. Slowly pull bar down behind head, pulling elbows in a downward and backward direction. Do not strain neck forward. Remember to breathe.

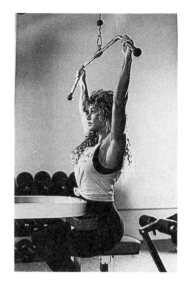

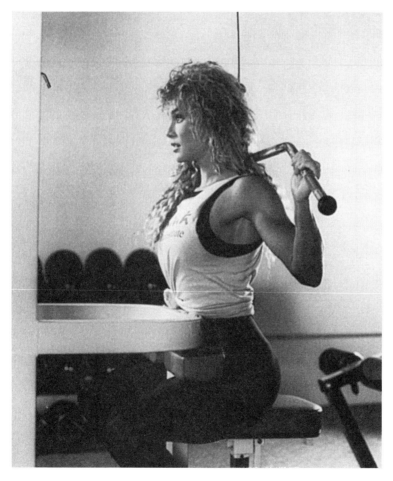

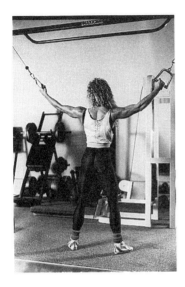

Shoulder retraction — Using high pulleys, stand with back straight and knees slightly bent. Slowly pull elbows in downward and backward direction behind back, squeezing shoulder blades together. Remember to breathe.

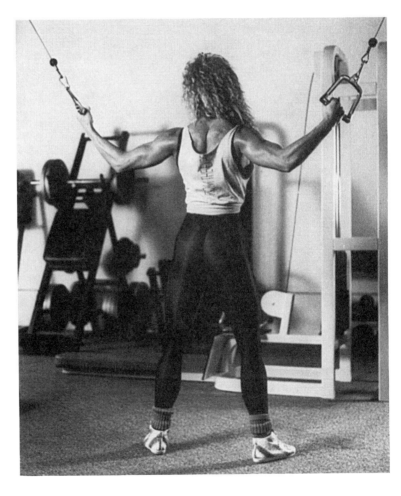

Low row — Sit upright with back straight and knees and hips bent. Keep feet shoulder width apart. Pull elbows backward, squeezing shoulder blades together. Return to starting position. Remember to breathe.

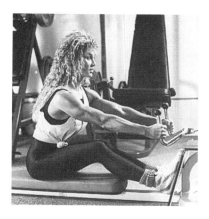

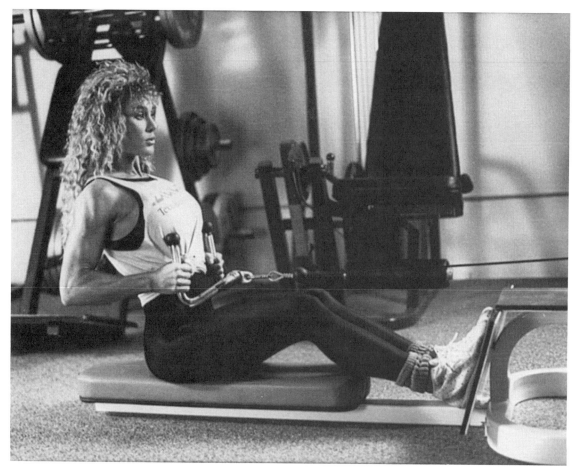

Free weights versus exercise machines

Generally speaking, a person with a back problem should avoid free weights initially. Exercise machines usually are safer. The range of motion used with weights can often be controlled better with a machine than with free weights.

In favor of free weights, however, we should point out that they build the stabilizer muscles of the trunk more than machines, mainly because the machine performs the task of balancing and stabilizing the weight for you.

We recommend that you start on machines, until you have developed enough strength to move into free weights later on.

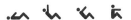

7

Sports and your back . . . or how not to hurt yourself while having fun

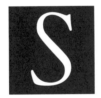ports are a great way to stay in shape. And there's a sport for every kind of person. Type A personalities, for example, may find sublime delight in mercilessly thrashing a helpless victim in a game of tennis, while type Bs may enjoy the serenity of a lone run through a quiet park.

If you're starting out in a sport, or if you're just interested in maximizing your lifelong back health in your current sport, here are some considerations to keep in mind.

Swimming

In addition to a great aerobic workout, the motions involved in swimming provide excellent shoulder and upper body strengthening. Another benefit of swimming is that water can make the body seem almost weightless. There is no jarring or bouncing on the spine, as in jogging or tennis. Impact injuries and muscle tears are rare from swimming.

Swimming raises certain concerns, however. The

crawl and breast stroke can force the back to hyperextend or arch backward, which — for some individuals — can cause lower back pain. Usually this can be avoided with the side-stroke or backstroke. The crawl can be acceptable as long as you use proper form. The body should be level as it pushes through the water with the head straight ahead rather than arched back.

Perhaps one of the most vulnerable areas of the body is where the mobile part of the neck connects to the immobile part of the thoracic spine. Neck pain can sometimes be caused by the sudden jerking of the head backward for a quick breath between strokes. In most cases, the repetitive nature of these motions creates an overuse syndrome.

Neck discomfort can be prevented by letting the body roll slightly on its side so that the head need only rotate rather than jerk backward. The key is to remember to keep the head going forward, rather than flicking it backward.

One sure solution to this problem is to use a snorkel. By breathing through the snorkel, the head stays perfectly level and moves straight ahead. It takes some practice to learn to use it, but it's well worth the trouble.

Neck discomfort can also occur when the swimmer changes the intensity or duration of the workout. Over time, however, the muscles will strengthen and adapt to the new level.

Sometimes swimming with a life vest will allow sufficient range of motion and further unweight the body in the water. A life vest is also an added safety precaution.

Ironically, swimmers can be susceptible to back injury because although they develop great upper body, arm, and leg strength, their backs remain relatively weak. Consequently, they may lift and wrestle with heavy objects that their backs are poorly trained to handle. Their backs are a weak link in an otherwise strong chain. The obvious solution to this problem is to balance swimming with exercises that specifically work the back.

Is swimming good for back pain? It depends. As noted in earlier chapters, hydrotherapy is a great way to ease back into activity. A warm pool can be therapeutic, and water creates an artificial weightlessness. For the person recovering from back pain, walking through the water is great. The water creates a heavy but subtle resistance to the legs and body.

Whether the person with back pain should try swimming depends greatly on individual swimming ability and form. Some people swim as though they are frantically trying to find a life raft. In such a case, swimming can worsen a preexisting problem.

Bicycling

Bicycling is a good overall conditioner because it improves aerobic and muscular endurance, especially in the legs. The only disadvantage of bicycling is that there is limited conditioning of the back muscles. In some cases, there may be flexion of the back, which could lead to back pain. And if the seat is too high and the handlebars are too low, it could cause your neck to arch backward, which can create an ache in the neck.

The bike must be set up properly for your body. There are five basic adjustments in fitting a bike to a rider: frame size, seat height, seat position, handlebar height, and reach.

Frame size — Today's bikes are much lighter and stronger than bikes made a decade ago. Frames may be made of chrome-magnesium alloys, aluminum or carbon fiber compositions. They may likewise differ in their ability to absorb shock from the roadway. When fitting the bike frame to the person, there should be at least one to two inches of space between the top tube and the rider's crotch when the rider straddles the bike with both feet flat on the ground.

Seat height — Saddle height is defined as the distance from the top of the seat to the center of the axis of the pedal spindle. With the pedal at the bottom of its arc, the rider's leg should almost be able to straighten out completely. Ideally, the leg should be bent only about 10 to 15 degrees at the knee.

Seat position — Seat position can be determined by placing the pedals in the three and nine o'clock positions, with the balls of the feet centered on the pedals. From this position, a plumb line dropped from the kneecap of the forward leg should line up with the center of the pedal. In other words, the kneecap of the forward leg should be right over the pedal. If it is not, slide the seat forward or back accordingly. The level of the seat should be horizontal, or angled so that the front part is slightly upward.

Handlebar height — The handlebars should be adjusted so that they are level with or just below the top of the seat.

Reach — Handlebar reach is the distance from the front tip of the saddle to the horizontal part of the handlebar. Place your elbow against the tip of the saddle. The tips of your extended fingers should just touch the handlebar. If this distance is way off, you may have to replace the stem of the handlebar with one having a different offset.

The type of bike used will determine how comfortable cycling will be for your back. The traditional racing-style bike, with low drop handlebars, may be super for low wind resistance, but the bent-over posture it requires places great strain on your back and neck. To see the road, for instance, the neck is continually arched backward.

A newer style of bike, often called a mountain bike, has straight handlebars and a frame that allows the rider to sit more upright. An added benefit is that this bike, thanks to bigger tires, does a better job of soaking up road shock. It is also a safer bike to ride because the wider tires provide better traction and stability than narrow racing tires — especially on pavement that is either wet or covered by loose sand or stones.

Running

Running gives the heart and legs an excellent workout. The back muscles are worked to a limited degree in holding the body upright. The only negative associated with running is that it has a jarring effect from the person's body weight continually hitting the ground. This impact sometimes affects joints and discs, causing temporary discomfort.

You can lessen this impact by investing in top-quality cushioned track shoes and by running on grass or a padded track. Also, shorter, more frequent runs are preferable to long marathon runs. As noted in the last chapter, there are benefits to "running forward" rather than at a slow jog, which places great up-and-down stress on the spine.

It's important in running to progress gradually to prevent injury. Never increase distance and pace simultaneously. Also, try to vary your cadence during a run to decrease the effects of constant, unvaried vibration.

People with existing back pain who wish to get into running should try wearing special lumbar support corsets as well as strengthening the abdominal muscles, which also support the lower back. Generally speaking, running can be a good way to maintain aerobic fitness and enjoy all the benefits of the body's own painkillers and mood enhancers.

Bodybuilding

One visit to a gym will convince you that bodybuilding, or body "shaping" as some call it, is a sport of the nineties. Once the domain of football players and male jocks, weight lifting has caught on with women. And for good reason: lifting weights not only improves performance at other sports, but also tones and makes for a more beautiful body.

Depending on how vigorously you pursue bodybuilding, the sport is a great way to selectively build up your resistance to body injury. Again, moderation is the best advice. Gymnasts typically have beautifully toned bodies, yet their emphasis is on flexibility and repetitive exercise rather than lifting heavy weights.

The greatest risks to bulking up relate to abusing heavy weights. Trying to lift more than you can handle can create a stress fracture, muscle strain, or ligament damage. In fact, weight lifters can be prone to spondylolysis, a stress fracture of the weak part of a lumbar vertebra in the spine. A good rule of thumb for back health in bodybuilding is to use lighter weights with higher repetitions, instead of lifting weights that you can lift only four to six times in succession.

The easiest way to injure your back in weight lifting is to perform extension/flexion exercises that arch your back against resistance. Simply put, avoid bending and lifting and bending and twisting exercises with heavy weight. The most risky moves for your back are the clean-and-jerk, the snatch, the squat, and dead-lift. All of these lifts force the back up in a hyperextended, or arched, position. If you are a serious bodybuilder, remember to take your time warming up, lift weights within your limit, always have someone spot you, and wear a weight belt to help support your lower back.

Age should also be a consideration in the intensity of your workouts. Although we can outwardly hide the signs of aging, internally, the discs in the spine begin drying and deteriorating as early as the teen years. The greatest degeneration occurs between 25 and 35 — the years when many weight lifters are lifting peak loads. By age 40, 80 percent of men and 65 percent of women have moderate disc degeneration. Interestingly, the extent of disc degeneration is even higher in weight lifters, even though they are stronger overall.

If you're serious about weight lifting, be careful about exercises that either stress the facet joints of the back or compress discs. Instead of performing standing squats with free weights to build up your legs, for example, use a machine that allows you to sit and press up the weight with your legs. Back exercises that encourage back flexibility should also be done on a daily basis. And of course, be sure to warm up thoroughly with stretches before starting any workout.

Lastly, if you don't already have a lifting belt, consider buying one. Why? Because it will probably help you prevent a back injury. How? That's something that back specialists are currently studying.

There are conflicting studies, for example, on the merits of lifting belts. Preliminary studies done at the Texas Back Institute show that lifting belts do appear to increase lifting strength. It's theorized that physiologically such lifting belts support abdominal musculature and decrease the pressure placed on the discs in the back during the lift.

Some experts, however, think that, over time, lifting belts may become a crutch. The lifting muscles themselves may fail to develop, setting up the back for injury when the belt is not on. Others theorize that the belts work psychologically. Because people feel support around the back, they try to lift more.

The Texas Back Institute recommends lifting belts for its patients and for workers in labor-intensive jobs. Theories aside, the physicians at the Texas Back Institute all agree on one important function of lifting belts: They remind someone to take care of his or her back. For that reason alone, a lifting belt will probably help prevent back injury.

Skiing

The risk of back injury goes up with sports that can abruptly twist or jerk the spine. Horseback riding, downhill skiing, dirt biking, water skiing, and powerboating across a rough lake are examples of how certain sports can have a jackhammer effect on the spine. In most cases, however, risk is related to a person's conditioning, with the out-of-shape weekend athlete having the highest risk of injury.

Skiing presents special risks because most people are not physically trained for falling either at the end of a tow rope or down a mountain. In addition to back injuries, for example, the ski patrols see a flurry of broken legs, ankles, and twisted knees every winter.

Except for those lucky enough to live in a mountain state, downhill skiing is limited to two or three weekends a year — definitely not enough to condition oneself to the high altitudes, the aerobic demands of the sport, the burst of muscular activity, and the trauma of falling down mountains. Never mind having to lug heavy skis and boots from the ski lodge to the car to the mountain, and then at the end of the day, lug it all back from the mountain to the car to the lodge when you're dead tired.

Consequently, skiers should begin conditioning programs at least six weeks before their outing. One of the best training exercises for skiing is the pillow jump. Place a pillow on the floor and practice jumping with both feet, sideways, from one side to the other. This exercise helps to strengthen your legs and knees by simulating the turning motions you perform with skis. After a few minutes you'll find it also builds aerobic endurance.

A good isometric exercise for skiers is to lower your back against a wall, as if you were sitting on a chair. Keep your feet body width apart and your heels about two feet away from the wall. Lower your body until your thighs are parallel with the floor. Hold for as long as you can without discomfort. Over a period of days, try to increase the time. This exercise does an excellent job of toning those thigh muscles, which you'll need on the slopes. If this exercise is too painful or rough on your knees, seriously reconsider why you're going skiing in the first place. Your body is giving you a loud warning to turn back now.

Unlike other sports where back strain is often the biggest danger, the inherent risk to the back from skiing is from falling. By skiing on slopes within one's ability, and by skiing in control, a person can limit much of the risk from snow skiing and still have fun.

The twisty sports: golf and tennis

Golf is a sport you can enjoy your entire life, even into old age. If that's your plan, invest the time now to learn proper golfing form from a pro. He or she will help you tap power from the correct transfer of weight and proper wrist release — as well as from coiling the back and shoulders. Lee Trevino, a former patient of the Texas Back Institute, and Fuzzy Zoeller are two touring pros who earn a good living despite serious back problems. The proper form helps.

The same advice applies to tennis. A survey of 143 players on the men's professional tennis tour showed that 38 percent had missed at least one tournament because of low back pain. John McEnroe, Tracy Austin, and Miroslav Mecir are just a few of the many famous tennis pros who have back problems.

Many back, tennis elbow, and shoulder problems stem from the high degree of body rotation and extension required to play tennis competitively. The tennis serve, in particular, forces the spine to hyperextend, which can temporarily compress the shock-absorbing discs between the vertebrae. The forehand, backhand, and volley similarly all require great amounts of trunk rotation to generate powerful tennis shots. All of these motions can become difficult as the player gets older and the discs in the spine become less resilient.

Older tennis players face obvious risks, but those younger players who attempt to become competitive at the game may also be at special risk. Some tennis experts have observed that over the years, tennis has evolved from a game that once prized grace and form to one that now emphasizes overpowering the opponent with brute force. Consequently, it is common for a junior competitor to undergo extremely long practice sessions, which can in turn cause fatigue and subsequent injury.

Similarly, tennis equipment has changed dramatically in recent years. In the seventies, tennis was played with wooden racquets, which were flexible and easy on the arm. In the eighties, stiffer metal and graphite rackets replaced wood. At the same time, tennis elbow and shoulder strains flourished. In the nineties, most new rackets are engineered with wide profiles to make them extremely stiff and powerful — but at a premium cost to the arm that swings them.

With any sport, consult a pro about equipment and how it may increase your chance of strain or injury. While you're in the pro shop, set up a lesson and have the pro check your form. Proper form can limit the stress on your body. Spend the time and money to learn form that will make you better at your sport without placing extraordinary demands on the back, or other parts of your body.

This chapter provides advice for some of the more common sports. Generally speaking, if your sport involves bending, twisting, lifting, or impact, the back is bound to be at risk. That doesn't mean you shouldn't enjoy the sport; just be aware that the risks need to be managed and controlled.

Good advice for all sports is to raise your heart rate gradually while warming up to increase your overall circulation. This will improve blood flow to tissues, especially in the back, and loosen stiff muscles and ligaments. Next, incorporate a brief stretching routine for your back which includes slowly bending, twisting, and extending backward. Lastly, slowly work up to full speed at the activity required in your sport.

Instead of heading from the car to the first tee with driver in hand, golfers should start on the practice range with short irons and slowly work up to a full swing with a driver. Then head for the first tee.

With tennis, rally with your opponent for at least 15 minutes, making sure you hit practice serves and overheads as well, before beginning your match.

And skiers, make one run down the green slope before heading to the top of the mountain and the double black trails.

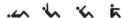

8

Making your job and home a back-friendly environment

he Texas Back Institute consults with many companies that are interested in reducing on-the-job injuries. In most cases, the task involves reviewing accident loss reports to see if certain jobs account for a high percentage of back injuries. If so, the job may be redesigned ergonomically to cause fewer injuries, or workers may be trained in safer ways of getting the job done without hurting their backs.

On one particular project, consultants from the Texas Back Institute were trying to help a waste management company lower its incidence of back injury. As we noted earlier, garbage collectors face the highest occupational risk of back injury because they perform the two most difficult jobs for the spine: lifting and twisting.

At first, the consultant looked at the design of the rear opening of the garbage trucks, the height of the opening, and other factors to see if the lifting and throwing distance required of each lifter could be lessened. Next she followed the workers around and watched how they lifted the bags.

After careful thought it appeared that short of massive job redesign, there were two ways to alter the job. First, she thought, why not lessen the weight of the bags that workers had to lift?

But unlike other companies that can design the size of their packages, garbage collectors have to deal with whatever is left for them. In fact, the supervisor noted, they had requested several times that customers limit the weight of each bag they filled, but the regulations were never observed, or at least not for long. People continued to stuff as much as possible into lawn-size plastic bags, drag them down to the end of the driveway, and let them sit.

Plan B was for workers to hold the load closer to their bodies while lifting to reduce stress on the spine. Seemed logical, until they asked her to try it herself. One smell was enough.

The point of this story is that there are limits to how easy you can make a particular task. No matter how well the job is designed, or how safe the worker is, there will always be risk of back injury.

The key is to eliminate needless risk. And just looking around your work place or home, you'll notice plenty of things that can be improved and made safer.

Ergonomics: The science of design

The word *ergonomics* is used more and more in today's work environment. In the most basic terms, ergonomics means trying to fit the job to the person instead of making the person fit the job.

The long-standing practice has been to design the dimensions of chairs, tables, desks and other tools and tasks to fit an average-sized person. Unfortunately, if you're a four-eleven woman or a six-six man, you know all too well what it feels like to sit in a car designed for the average-sized person. The woman may find that if she moves up the seat to reach the pedals, the steering wheel may feel too close. The man, on the other hand, may find his head brushes the roof.

Thankfully, recognition of the factor of human individuality is beginning to find its way into car engineering and work station design. In real life, as we all know, no two people are exactly alike, and there are real benefits to engineering a comfortable and safe car, or designing a work station that yields the greatest productivity for a variety of different workers.

As it relates specifically to the back, ergonomics plays an important role in maintaining spine alignment and reducing the fatigue experienced in the back and neck over time or with repetition of various movements. Here are some ways you can make your work place and home a better and safer environment for your back:

Finding a chair that fits

Sure, everyone knows that you can strain your back when lifting. But did you know that you can strain your back when sitting?

Interestingly, sitting has been found to be a key contributor to back injury in many people.

Because sitting does not involve heavy or repetitive work, it has often been overlooked as a cause of back trouble. Logically, one would think that by sitting, the back is given a chance to relax. But actually, sitting is a static posture, which can add a tremendous amount of pressure to the back muscles and discs. Just as poor posture can wear down the back's resistance to injury over time, sitting can set the back up for injury.

Sitting in a slouched-over or slouched-down position creates excessive flexion, overstretches the spinal ligaments, and increases disc pressure. Sitting with the back relatively straight minimizes the load on the back. Add an ergonomically designed chair and the back is supported even better at its weakest area — the low back area. Also, an ergonomically designed chair makes it difficult and uncomfortable to slouch; it seems to make you want to sit right.

Consequently, if you spend eight hours a day sitting, invest in a good chair. If you can't get your company to buy it, and if you don't want to buy it yourself, get a portable orthopedic insert. Or at least roll up a towel to help support the low back in midposition.

What's a good chair and how do you find one that's just right for you? Here are some tips:

The seat pad — The seat pad should not put pressure on the backs of the knees. It should be short enough to allow a few inches of space behind the knee area. This prevents pressure from being placed on the blood vessels and nerves that pass through that area. The seat pad width should provide space on either side of the body for motion and comfort, but should not be so wide that it lacks support.

The arm rests — The arm rests should be close enough so that you do not have to lean to the side to reach them. It is best if the arm rests are adjustable.

The seat back — The seat back is critical, because it is the one part of the chair that your back will spend the most time leaning against. The seat back should be able to tilt backward about 10 degrees. This helps take some pressure off the back. The height of the seat back should correspond to the height of the person to give the appropriate support to the back. Don't buy a chair that has a seat back that is too low to support the length of the back. The seat back must also be wide enough to support the back. If you have a broad back, keep this in mind. A good seat back should be slightly wider than the torso and allow lateral support with slightly curved sides. The seat back should also have enough tension to support the back and not fall too far backward. The good seat back should also have some type of lumbar support. Ideally, this feature should be adjustable so it can be customized for each person's back.

The seat frame — The chair should turn easily and, if

needed, have casters so you can roll around and change locations. You shouldn't have to jerk the chair to get it moving. Special plastic mats for chairs can also be purchased to make the chair mobile on a carpeted or rough surface.

Comfortable? Remember not to sit for too long. Get up and move around every hour or so to relax and recharge your muscles. It will be a relief to your back to enjoy a different position for a change.

Finding a comfortable work height

Look at the level where you'll be working. The bench height often isn't the best work height. The most common ergonomic mistakes seen in the work place are making workers perform tasks at improper work heights, requiring them to assume a static posture, asking them to perform repetitive motions, and assigning tasks that are too heavy.

In designing a standing work station, the work height should be high enough that you need not have to bend your neck to do your work on the table top. If the work height is too low, raise the table. If that is not possible, raise your work by elevating it upon several large boards or books.

At a sitting work station, the same guidelines apply. Adjust the chair to what feels like a comfortable height and position. If you work with a computer, elevate the monitor so that you don't need to raise and lower your head when looking at either the keyboard or the screen. Typically, the top of the screen should be at eye level. If the screen is too low, raise it up on several large books or another type of prop. Many computer stores routinely carry monitor stands for just such a reason.

How to stand

Many injuries happen due to the stresses of standing. It is very important to change your position every few minutes to give the muscles a break. Good techniques for relieving stress while standing are

- Using something to prop your foot up on to help rest back muscles
- Changing feet every few minutes to allow the stresses to be evened
- Wearing good-quality shoes that provide good arch support, as well as a good cushion. This is especially important if you work on hard concrete floors all day long.
- Using a cushioned floor covering if possible to help absorb shock; using throw rugs around the house on wooden floors if necessary
- Using a high chair or stool to sit on whenever possible to rest your legs and back

How to lift something close to your body

Next time you are near a construction site, look at the cranes that have the tough task of hoisting heavy girders and concrete. There are ground-level mobile cranes that resemble giant steam shovels and there are tall stationary cranes that resemble a giant letter T. The mobile crane usually has a main beam that stays relatively upright. In fact, it rarely lowers below a 45-degree angle because that lessens the leverage it is able to impart with its pulley.

The stationary crane, on the other hand, uses a different design to accomplish the same lifting task. The main lifting beam always remains parallel to the ground, and instead uses a large counterweight to create leverage.

The same techniques should be used when you have to lift something. Whenever you must lift something, always try to maneuver it as close as possible to your body. By keeping the object close to the body, not only are you reducing the strain on your spine, but you place the weight in a position where the powerful leg muscles can help out. In this example, you are acting like a ground-level crane.

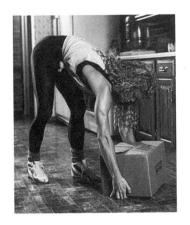

Left, the wrong way to lift. Below are two different ways that do not strain the back. In the first example, Cory keeps her feet apart to provide a wide base of support. Next, she slides her fingers underneath the box. She then raises the object to mid-thigh, keeping it close to the body, and begins to stand, using the power of the leg muscles. As she stands, she gradually straightens her back the rest of the way. At no time is the back completely bent over. In the bottom example, Cory starts with one knee on the floor, raises the box to mid-thigh, and then stands. Remember: use your legs to lift, not your back.

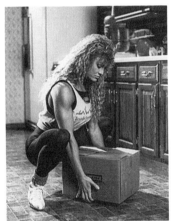
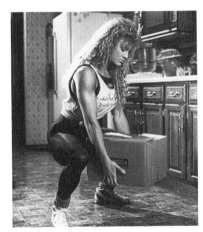
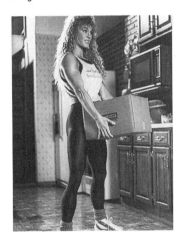

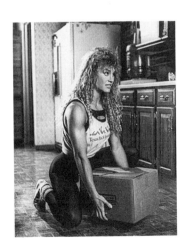
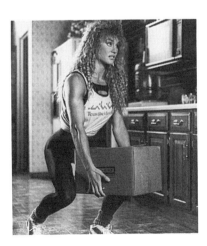
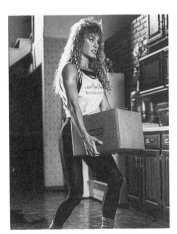

How to lift something you can't get close to

Sometimes you are not able to move the object close to the body. A good example is when you have to lean into the back seat of a car to take a squirming baby out of a safety seat. Lifting golf clubs, groceries or luggage out of the trunk of a car can also present special problems.

To lift something out of the back seat, brace yourself by placing one knee on the seat. To lift something out of the trunk, the bumper may provide a brace. If neither the seat nor bumper on your car can be used, extend one of your legs backward, which will act as a counterweight as you stretch outward. In this sense, you will be lifting like a stationary crane, which uses a counterweight to lift.

Is it better to push or pull?

If you have a choice, which is easier on your back — pushing or pulling an object? If you must move something, pushing is less stressful than pulling.

When pulling, there is too much opportunity to jerk, which in turn may strain muscles or, worse, herniate a disc. Also, most of the weight must be pulled by the back muscles. When pushing, however, the weight is moved more by the powerful leg muscles than by the back.

Driving long distances

If your car doesn't have ergonomically designed seats, find a lumbar support for your low back, or roll up a towel and place it in the small of the low back.

Unlike sitting behind a desk, sitting in a car imparts a constant vibration to the spine. Over the course of a long drive, this can tire the back, which has been trying to absorb the vibration. Truck drivers, not surprisingly, often have back pain as a by-product of their long hauls.

A good habit is to stop every hour and walk around a rest area. Do some standing stretches — forward, backward and side to side — to refresh the muscles.

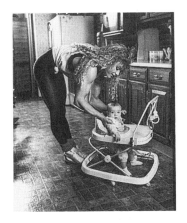

Left, the wrong way to wrestle your baby out of a stroller. The back is at extreme risk because the infant often will get a foot stuck as he or she is being lifted clear of the stroller.

Below are two correct ways. In the first example, Cory kneels down and raises baby out of the stroller and to her chest. Then she merely has to stand, using the power of the leg muscles. In the bottom example she squats, keeping her back straight, and uses her arms rather than her back to hoist baby up and away from the stroller. Always avoid twisting when lifting.

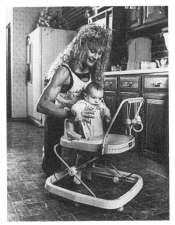
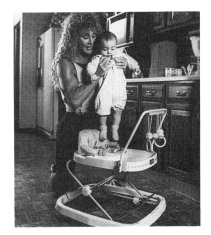
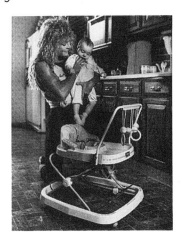
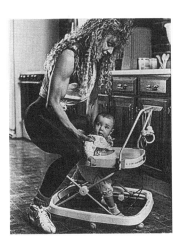
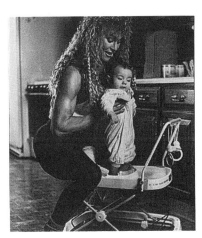
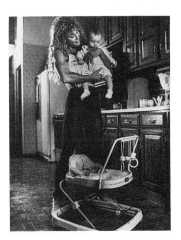

Perhaps the worst thing to do after a long drive is to park and then jerk your luggage out of the trunk. Your back is fatigued and not ready to lift a loaded suitcase while you are bent over at the waist. A better idea might be to have dinner or a drink, walk around the hotel a little, and then worry about the luggage. Even better: have a hotel employee, or your host, help with the luggage.

Whether you are sitting, standing, or walking, ergonomic principles can apply to everyone at home and work. Think about your daily activities in both settings. Do you have any recurring or consistent aches and pains? Do you usually spend a lot of time in one position or posture? Do you have difficulty handling or reaching for anything?

Lastly, remember that solutions don't have to involve costly changes. Use what is on hand whenever possible, if it is safe. You don't have to rebuild all the cabinets in your home, for instance, if they are too high. Instead, get a step stool and stop straining to reach the higher items.

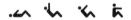

PART III

What If You Already Have Back Pain?

9

Home remedies for back pain

T ake two aspirins and call me in the morning. For someone suffering from an attack of excruciating back pain, it's understandable to expect more from a visit to the doctor. Hard as it is to believe, however, because most back pain is related to muscle strain, taking anti-inflammatories like aspirin or ibuprofen and getting off your feet is still good advice.

Nurses at the Texas Back Institute who answer the Back Pain Hotline (1-800-247-BACK) often recommend that and other home remedies for individuals whose symptoms imply a simple strain. At the same time, they caution that if the back pain doesn't get better with anti-inflammatories over a period of one to three days, it could be a sign that the person needs to make the trip to a back specialist to get checked out.

The Back Pain Hotline at the Texas Back Institute doesn't diagnose medical problems—no one can do that over the phone — but it does provide quick answers to those suffering an attack of back pain. Even simple muscle strain can cause the type of sharp pain that can make someone panic.

It's common for people to call the hotline in a breathless panic, fearing that they have herniated discs or fractured vertebrae and now may need surgery to stop the pain. In a few instances, there are individuals who have symptoms — like loss of control of the bowel or bladder — that imply serious spinal cord impingement. And these people are instructed to seek out either a spine surgeon or hospital emergency room for immediate care. In most cases, however, the symptoms imply a mild strain that can be treated at home.

This in a sense is another key function of the Back Pain Hotline — to save people money. Each year, it's estimated that Americans spend $16 billion on back pain. The reason why the hotline nurses often recommend that a person wait a day or so before seeking out a doctor is because most back pain will go away on its own.

The other reason is that unless you go to a back specialist, there may be little real benefit versus the cost. If the physician does not have a team of physical therapists who are trained in back care, for example, his or her options will be limited to prescribing just anti-inflammatories, muscle relaxers, and bed rest. People are saddened to learn that doctors have no magic wands.

Yet going to the doctor does make sense, because the physician may be able to rule out if you have done any serious damage to your back and perhaps more clearly diagnose what may be causing your back pain attack. For some back pain sufferers, this peace of mind can be worth 100 times the cost of a physician visit.

Also, if you go to a back specialist, chances are that specialized physical therapy will be prescribed for you which can relieve the episode of back pain. The therapists will also give you a customized exercise program that will recondition your muscles and help prevent a recurrence of back strain.

Danger signals: When to see a doctor

As noted earlier, most simple back pain will start to improve with a day or two of rest and taking aspirin. If you find that you're taking more and more pills to relieve back pain, or if the pain is getting worse, head for a back specialist.

Foot drop, where the person drags a foot because the leg muscles cannot raise the toes, is a sign of a serious neurological problem such as nerve impingement or a ruptured disc. Another extremely serious signal is loss of bowel or bladder control. A person with these symptoms should go immediately to a spine specialist or a hospital emergency room. If you ignore signals like these, the loss of muscular control over these parts of the body could become permanent.

Pain that radiates down an arm or leg implies that a nerve is being pinched — perhaps from a bulging or ruptured disc. A ruptured disc doesn't necessarily require surgery to repair it. At the Texas Back Institute, for example, most patients with ruptured discs recover from their back pain without surgery. Often, the problem of a herniated disc can be treated successfully through a combination of rest, medicine, injections and an exercise program that strengthens the supporting muscles and ligaments in the back.

Still interested in doing it yourself? If so, here's an effective first-aid guide for a simple back attack.

Home remedy #1: Stop what you're doing

It's hard to believe, but some golfers will hurt their backs on the second hole yet continue to play until putting out on the last green. If you think you've hurt your back, you are much better off stopping immediately.

Many others have no choice in the matter. Their back pain will literally force them to drop to their knees. Others will be frozen bent over. Either way, back pain is a signal to stop what you're doing.

For years, bed rest has been a common treatment for back injury. In the past, it wasn't unusual for a doctor to tell a patient to remain at bed rest for weeks, even months. But recent research has shown that prolonged bed rest is actually more harmful than it is helpful. In fact, studies on acute back pain show that two days of bed rest is as good as a week or more in allowing the strained muscles to unbind and relax. In most episodes of simple back pain the person begins to feel better on his own after a couple days.

When bed rest and anti-inflammatories don't help you within a day or so, however, you should seek out a back specialist, because this is often a sign that something more serious is wrong.

To get the most out of only two days of bed rest, completely unload the spine. Don't lie face down, for example, because this position still places some strain on your back. The position that best unloads all body weight is to lie on the back with a pillow under the knees. The second best position is on the side with a pillow between the knees.

Next, read magazines, do office work, a crossword puzzle or watch television — anything to distract your mind from the pain signal it is receiving.

Home remedy #2: Aspirin or ibuprofen

As explained in earlier chapters, back pain may arise from irritated muscles, ligaments, facet joint capsules, a swollen disc, or inflamed and irritated nerves. Anti-inflammatories are thought to be effective in reducing swelling.

Of all the nonprescription drugs, acetaminophen, aspirin and the ibuprofen products like Advil, Nuprin, and Medipren have become the most commonly used anti-inflammatories. Acetaminophen-based medications like Tylenol or Datril act as an analgesic and antipyretic to reduce pain and fever. Acetaminophen is perhaps a little better at relieving pain than aspirin, but then aspirin has more anti-inflammatory properties which can be useful in reducing swelling in muscle-related back pain. Essentially, acetaminophen has the least anti-inflammatory effect, while ibuprofen has more anti-inflammatory effect but less analgesic effect than acetaminophen. And aspirin is somewhere in the middle. In general, the best medication for home first aid would be either aspirin or ibuprofen.

Some brands of aspirins, like Ecotrin or Encaprin, are enteric-coated to prevent stomach irritation. This coating can help the pills withstand the acids in the stomach so they can be broken down later by the enzymes in the intestines. Bufferin and Ascriptin, on the other hand, contain ingredients like those in Maalox to make the aspirin less acidic and lessen the stomach irritation. But that's not as proven as the enteric-coating approach. If your stomach hurts 10 minutes after taking an aspirin, you should consider taking an enteric-coated aspirin or ibuprofen.

Remember, these medications are more effective if you begin taking them right after the injury occurs. Also, never take medication on an empty stomach. Take these medications after a meal and at bedtime with a glass of milk.

As for dosage, you should always take the smallest dosage that relieves pain, up to the manufacturer's limit listed on the box. Overmedicate yourself and you'll regret it. Virtually every medicine has a side effect. Overdosing on an acetaminophen product can have a side effect on a person's liver. In extreme cases, it can cause irreversible liver damage. Aspirin, in fact, is the most commonly overdosed drug in the United States. People, especially those with arthritis, take increasing amounts of aspirin to relieve their pain. Ultimately, overdosing on aspirin can alter blood gases, which could, in the worst case, cause a coma. A less acute side effect is that some people have gastric problems, such as ulcers in the stomach, from aspirin. Overdosing on ibuprofen, likewise, causes gastric problems.

Home remedy #3: Ice, then heat

Remember this rule: ice first for 48, then heat.

Ice and heat are both effective in helping to alleviate some of the local pain that comes from muscle and ligament strain. Heat will increase the blood flow to the deep tissues, whereas ice will act as a local anesthetic and prevent swelling. Both extreme heat or cold can hurt the skin if they are left directly on the skin for more than five minutes at a time. Research has proven that ice slows the swelling and inflammation that occurs after injury. It also acts as an anesthetic by numbing sore tissues. After 48 hours, however, ice has lost its effect. Using heat thereafter is thought to aid the healing process by increasing circulation and relaxing muscle spasms.

Here's a great first-aid tip: Take several paper cups and fill them almost to the top with water. Then put them in the freezer. When frozen, peel the edge of the cup back one inch and have someone gently apply the ice cup to the area of soreness on the back. Lie on your stomach with a pillow under your hips or lie on your side and apply the ice in a circular motion over a six-inch area where you feel the pain, but avoid the area directly over the spine. Massage the area with the ice for about five minutes at a time.

Essentially, the cold will make the veins in the tissue contract, reducing circulation. Then once you stop applying cold, the veins overcompensate and dilate, allowing blood to rush into the sore area. This blood, along with the oxygen it carries, will begin healing the damaged tissue.

This treatment is common for sports injuries. On the sidelines you'll see a football player with an ice pack on a sore knee, for example. Thereafter, he may switch and rest the joint in a warm whirlpool bath. Your own bathtub at home is just as good.

Home remedy #4: Massage

If you have a willing companion, gentle massage may provide some temporary relief by stretching out tight muscles and ligaments.

As a side note: while massage is okay for a sore back, don't incorporate massage into your first-aid technique for newly injured arms or legs. Stick with ice and heat.

Home remedy #5: Exercise

Probably the most beneficial remedy for back pain is exercise. This is ironic, in a sense, because when one suffers from back pain, just the word *exercise* can be enough to make one wince.

In reality, there have been numerous studies that maintain that exercise is more effective at treating simple back pain than passive methods such as rest and drugs. There are several reasons.

First, exercise narrows the source of pain to a smaller area. Exercise, in fact, is the best way to centralize the pain from a broad area to a localized area, reduce pain, accelerate the healing process, and lastly prevent the injury from happening again.

And that is exactly the kind of result the Texas Back Institute is after with its unique treatment program. Those who take their back pain to the Texas Back Institute are amazed to see a clinic that looks more like a health club than a repository for the nation's worst cases of back pain. The Texas Back Institute is both. People start off with disability, but end up with ability.

Second, exercise stimulates the body's production of its own natural painkillers, called endorphins and enkephalins. Without exercise, the production of endorphins and other mood enhancers falls off dramatically. One must make exercise part of a daily routine for both the painkilling benefits as well as for maintaining strength and endurance.

Home exercises that relieve back pain

The following pages illustrate several exercises that are effective at relieving back pain. Consider these first-aid exercises. They are intended to restore the lordosis, or natural curve, to the low back, as well as improve flexibility and lessen stiffness.

The first extension exercise shown, the press-up, is an important exercise for relieving simple back pain. This exercise has been championed over the years by Robin MacKenzie, a New Zealand physical therapist. MacKenzie was one of the first back specialists to document the effectiveness of extension exercises through several studies. Consequently, his name has become synonymous with these exercises.

Flexion exercises, on the other hand, were pioneered 40 years ago by a Texas orthopedic surgeon, Dr. Paul Williams. For years, it was common for back specialists to prescribe Williams's flexion exercises for back pain sufferers.

Over the years, the Texas Back Institute has found that a combination, or selection, of extension and flexion exercises produces the best results after a back pain attack.

A word of caution, however. It is impossible to prescribe a general, all-encompassing home remedy exercise program for all cases when people have various types of disc bulges, disc herniations, facet joint problems, or muscle strains. Here are some guidelines to consider before you start.

Muscle strain injuries and disc problems tend to respond better to extension exercises. Indeed, in some cases, flexion exercises may increase pain.

On the other hand, *those people with facet problems, for example, feel much better when they do flexion exercises* and worse when they do extension exercises.

The first important rule of thumb to follow, then, with these home remedy exercises is as follows: *If your back begins to hurt worse with a specific exercise, stop doing it.*

Find the exercises that make your back feel better and use those. Initially, there may be some discomfort with any of these exercises, especially if your back is extremely sore, and if before your injury you weren't used to exercising at all. For this type of inactive person, any type of exercise is going to be uncomfortable.

Some minor discomfort must be worked through before you can achieve the benefit from exercise. Only you can decide what is discomfort from inactivity and what is a level of pain signaling that your body is warning you to stop what you're doing.

Remember, these few exercises are only a means to an end. Once you have relief from your back pain, begin the back strengthening exercises shown earlier in the book.

Rule of thumb number two: A serious attack of back pain may cause pain that always seems present, whether sitting, standing or even lying down. It may feel even worse when you're moving from one position to another. *If you can't straighten up fully, or perform any of these first-aid exercises without severe pain, stick to bed rest. And if your pain is this disabling, this may be a signal to visit a back specialist to rule out any serious back injury.*

It should be noted that in the case of a large disc herniation, for example, certain exercises may actually make your pain worse. If you find this happening to you as you perform these exercises, you should visit a spine specialist for professional help. (See Chapter 10 to find the type of back specialist most experienced in dealing with herniated discs.)

The best exercise to start with is the press-up. It can be done several times a day, or whenever you sense an attack of pain returning. Again, if this extension exercise worsens your pain, skip to the flexion exercises.

In theory, all of these exercises attempt to recentralize the soft nucleus of the disc, which may have shifted backward toward the facet joints. By extending backward, the vertebrae may gently push the nucleus back into position and relieve the stress on nearby nerves.

The intent of flexion exercises is to restore flexibility. As with any exercise on a sore back, there may be some discomfort, but it should lessen with repetition of the exercise, which implies that the back is becoming more flexible.

If the pain begins to increase with each subsequent repetition, however, you should stop. It may be that flexion exercises are worsening your back problem.

The best number of repetitions for these home remedy exercises is between 10 and 30.

After completing these exercises, relax by lying on your back with a lumbar roll or a rolled-up towel supporting the curve in the low back. These exercises can also be done on a regular basis either in the morning or evening, or throughout the day when you feel stiffness or discomfort returning.

Another exercise that can help relieve back pain is walking — as long as your back pain doesn't get worse in the process. A stationary bike is also a good alternative.

Ideally, you want to break into a little sweat. This is the telltale sign that you are raising the temperature of the muscle tissues. The ultimate goal here is to get the heart pumping oxygen-rich blood to the site of the injury. It is felt that this fresh oxygen and the increase in tissue temperature will help relax muscles in spasm and quiet irritated nerves. Improved circulation is also the first step in helping the tissue to heal.

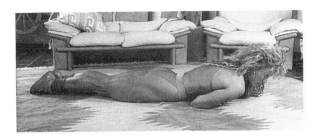

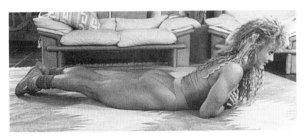

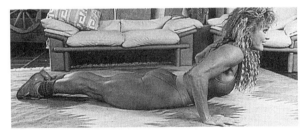

Extension exercise: Press-up — For the person in acute back pain, start by lying face down or on your elbows for three to five minutes.

For others, try using your arm strength to press up and back as far as possible. Hold for 10 seconds and repeat.

At first, your arms may have to be bent as you press up. Try to work up to where you can straighten your arms completely. The first few press-ups may be uncomfortable, but pain should lessen with subsequent sessions.

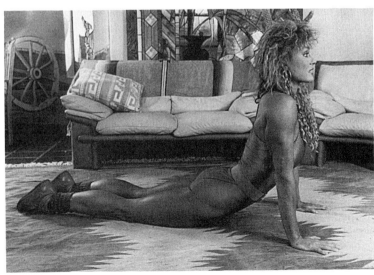

Flexion exercise:
Pelvic tilt — Lie on back with knees raised and arms extended. Press the low back down against the floor by tightening the abdominal muscles, squeezing buttocks and rolling top of pelvis backward. Hold for 10 seconds.

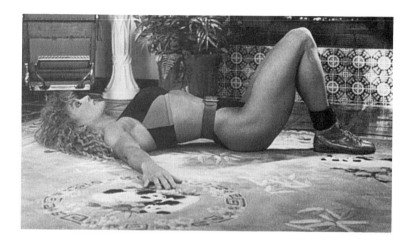

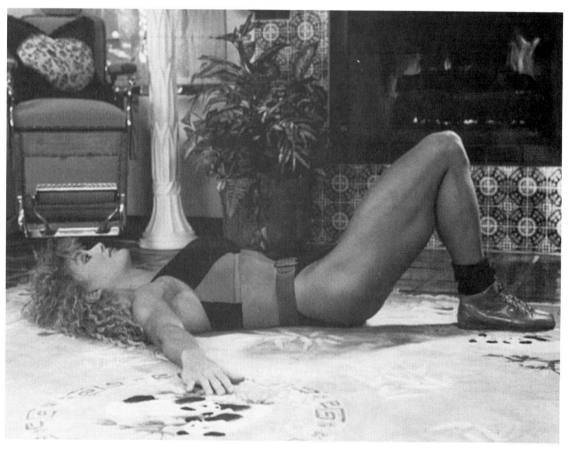

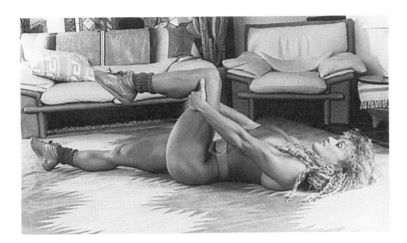

Flexion exercise:
Single knee to chest —
Lie on back and lift one
knee to chest. Repeat
with other leg. Hold for 10
seconds.

    Some people may
find flexion extremely
difficult immediately
after a back pain attack.
If so, gradually work into
this exercise.

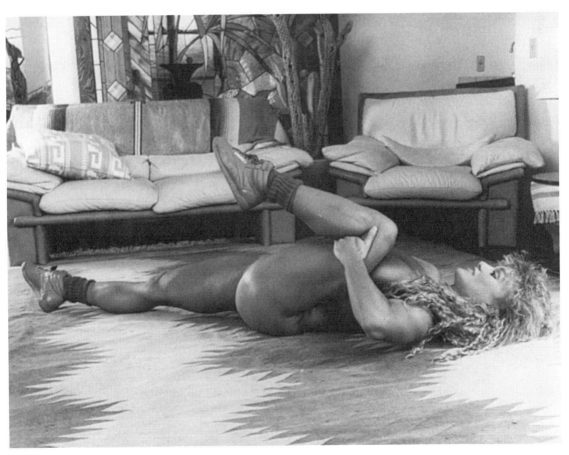

Flexion exercise: Double knee to chest — Lie on back, lift one knee and then the other to chest. Keep knees together. Hold for 10 seconds. Remember to keep your low back in contact with the floor. If you can, try to lift your head and touch your forehead to your knees.

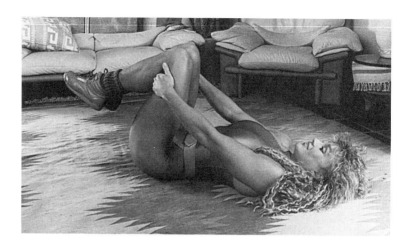

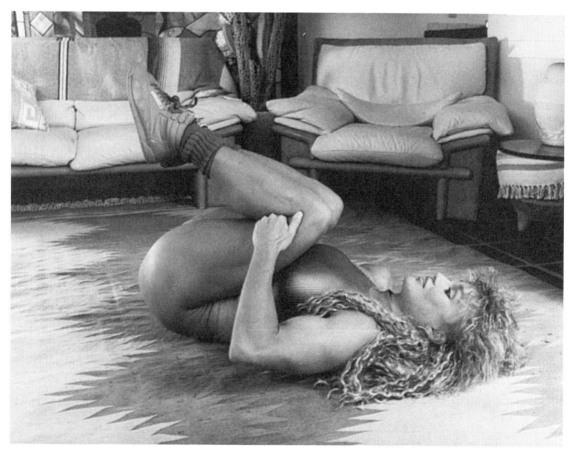

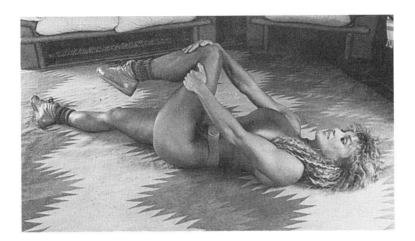

Flexion exercise: Piriformis stretch — Lie on back with one leg extended. Position other leg with knee bent and crossed over extended leg. Grasp behind bent knee and pull up and across toward opposite shoulder. Hold for 10 seconds.

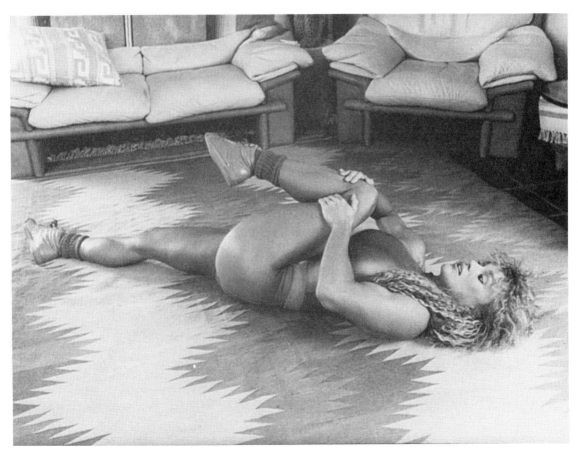

Extension and flexion
exercise: In a kneeling
position, arch your back
slowly downward, then
upward.

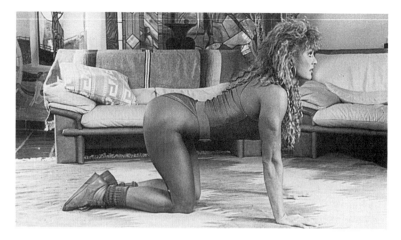

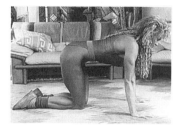

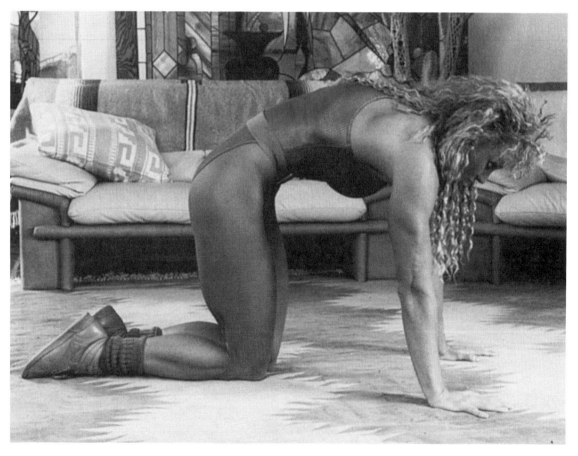

Home remedy #6: Adjust

When you are in pain, you will need to make some adjustments in your approach to your daily activities.

First, sit as little as possible and for short periods. Choose a chair that is firm with a straight back. Avoid soft, low furniture like sofas and use a lumbar roll or rolled-up towel to support the low back. When sitting down use your legs to lower to the front of the chair and then scoot back. To get up, scoot to the front of the chair and use your leg and arm power.

Drive as little as possible. If you must drive, make sure the driver's seat is in a position to support the back fully and that your arms are held straight out to the steering wheel. Bring your lumbar roll or rolled-up towel to fill in the low back area.

Avoid lifting anything heavy. And certainly avoid objects that are awkward to carry. Test the weight before you lift and hold the object close to you. Don't try to lift something over your head, and use your legs to lift anything from below the waist.

In bed, use pillows for positioning. Make sure your bed has a firm base and doesn't sag in the middle. When getting up, roll to your side, draw your knees up, push up to a sitting position and stand up by pushing up with your legs.

Home remedy #7: Relax your head

Biofeedback is an extension of the normal way in which we learn. Learning is a process of getting feedback through our eyes, ears, nose, and hands and connecting this new information for doing an activity again in the future. For example, when you swing your tennis racket, you feel your arm move, your wrist tighten, and your hand squeeze the grip. You observe your racket connecting with the tennis ball, and you feel your follow-through. Then you observe where the ball lands. If you're happy with the result, you'll try to reproduce the process on your next stroke.

What does all of this have to do with back or neck

pain? Medical evidence indicates that stress and depression can have a variety of effects on our bodies. Normally, most people calm down after a stressful event. But some others do not. They can stay keyed up for a long time afterward.

Back or neck pain is stressful. Our normal reaction is to protect the part of our body that is causing us pain. How do we protect it? By nature, we all are conditioned to tense the muscles that surround our back or neck. But such tension can increase back and neck pain, which leads to more tension. As you can see, back pain itself can create a vicious cycle of pain that begets tension that begets even more pain and even more tension. Because this is a habitual response, we often aren't even aware of this tension cycle. We just become victims of the symptoms that result.

Biofeedback technicians at the Texas Back Institute use sophisticated electronic equipment to give back pain sufferers insight into this process. Electrodes are attached to different muscle groups such as the frontalis (forehead) and trapezius (shoulder). The machine amplifies the sound of electrical activity in those muscle groups. People are surprised to learn that they are under great stress and tension as a by-product of their back pain. They are equally surprised to learn they can control and lessen this tension without drugs. This is accomplished by learning various relaxation techniques.

Some people may always suffer from residual back pain because of the nature of their back problem. Others may prefer to try to adjust to a small level of pain rather than attempt to remove it through surgery. In both cases, these back pain sufferers might normally have to rely on drugs to help them manage their back pain. Over time, however, this reliance on drugs may create a drug dependency, or show side effects on other functions of the body. Such persons are better off learning techniques that enable them to cope with their back pain without depending on drugs.

But relaxation techniques first have to be learned and then they must be continually practiced. There are many

benefits, however. Biofeedback
- relieves fatigue and lowers anxiety
- relieves pain of joints and muscles
- relieves insomnia
- lowers blood pressure
- allows quality rest
- helps one to cope better
- gives a sense of well-being

Autogenics or self-suggestion

Autogenic techniques are sometimes called mind over matter. In essence, your mind is telling your body how it should feel.

Lie in a nice warm bath. After you relax for a few minutes, say out loud to yourself, "My left arm feels heavy and warm." Repeat this several times. As you concentrate, try to feel your arm actually getting heavier and warmer. Really try. Then repeat the command, focusing on your right arm, left leg, and so on.

Guided imagery or visualization

One of the most exciting developments in the field of professional athletics is the concept of visualization. Some studies, for example, tested one group of basketball players who practiced shooting free throws for hours. Another group was not allowed to practice shooting free throws. Instead, the members of this group were trained to visualize themselves shooting free throws and having every single ball arch up perfectly and then down through the center of the hoop. When subsequently tested together, the visualization group improved to the same extent as the others who had spent their time actually practicing free throws.

Similarly, Olympic bobsledders spend hours visualizing the experience of traveling rapidly down through the course at high rates of speed. And professional tennis players routinely visit sports psychologists to learn how to maximize their performance in key tournaments.

Such mind power can be equally effective in helping you manage pain. While lying in a warm bath, imagine a beautiful, serene, tranquil place that you particularly like. Take a vacation in your mind to that place. Imagine it in detail — how it looks . . . smells . . . sounds . . . feels. Are there animals there? Do they make interesting sounds? Create a motion picture in your mind and don't leave a single thing out. If your ideal place is a beach at sunset, don't forget to add the sound of the crashing surf on the reef. Or the sound of the wind rustling through the palm trees overhead. Is the ocean breeze cold? If so, let it give you a noticeable chill as you think about it. Are there any other people in your dream? Are they good-looking? Well, you get the picture.

As you continue to get lost in the setting you've created for yourself, imagine how relaxed and peaceful you feel sitting in that place.

While a bath may help you get in the right frame of mind, this relaxation technique can be done anywhere. You might find it somewhat hard to explain to someone nearby why a silly little smile has crept across your face.

Start by finding a comfortable position, preferably sitting in a straight-back chair. There is a tendency to fall asleep if you lie down. Allow your mind to quiet by taking several slow, deep breaths. If your eyes are not already closed, close them now. Focus on the sensation of the air just inside the tip of your nose.

Breathe normally. On your first breath inhale, focusing just on sensations of air flowing by at the tip of your nose. As you exhale, continue to focus on these sensations and mentally count to yourself: "One."

Count each breath while focusing on these same sensations until you reach four, then start over again with one. Continue breathing in this fashion for about 10 minutes. If you lose count or your mind starts to wander, start over again with one.

This exercise produces a state of relaxation and develops concentration. The idea is not to force thoughts out of your mind, but simply to focus on your breathing. Although the goal is to increase your awareness and concentration while awake, you may want to do the exercise at night if you have difficulty falling asleep or if you wake up in the night.

Here is another relaxation technique that may be done while sitting or reclining in a chair or while lying on a bed, sofa, or the floor.

Close your eyes and begin by taking several minutes to concentrate on your breathing. Take several slow, deep breaths. Imagine exhaling tension and inhaling relaxation. Tense the muscles in one part of your body, beginning with your hands, and move from one muscle group to another, ending with your feet and finally tense your entire body.

Hold each position only four or five seconds. Pause and relax for 15 seconds after tensing each muscle group. Enjoy the relaxation. Once you can recognize tension in your body, it will be unnecessary to tense muscles voluntarily. Just locate the tension and let it go. To relax, you must be able to distinguish between tension and relaxation. Remember: the mind is like a muscle. If you exercise it with these drills, your concentration will be that much stronger and your ability to control pain and stress that much better. By increasing your control over voluntary muscles, you can consciously relax these muscles on command.

Home remedy #8: Sex

It's common for sex and recreation in general to take a back seat to one's recovery from back injury.

Sure, the regular bowling night and tennis game may have to be canceled while a person builds up back strength. If you are unable to walk or run without pain, then do a less strenuous activity. Playing cards, dominoes, Monopoly, Trivial Pursuit or one of many such games affords a good mental diversion.

The important point here is that recreation needs to be continued throughout recovery. Not only is recreation a great way to divert the brain's attention away from the pain signals it may be receiving from nerves, but it also promotes better overall mental health. When it comes to mental diversions, perhaps one of the best ones is sex.

Sex can be extremely important during a person's recovery from back pain. A question that is frequently avoided by patients recovering from serious back pain or back surgery is "When can I resume sexual activity?" For some, even talking about sex can be a source of embarrassment.

This is a perfectly normal question that a person should ask his or her physician. Many times a physician will automatically inform patients when they may resume sexual activity. Whether the patient asks or is told, the extent of the sexual activity must be self-controlled.

As with physical exercise, pain is generally the most common limiting factor with sex. When it comes to sex, however, there is an important mental component. If a patient fears a recurrence of a back pain attack, he or she might refrain from any sexual activity.

In the case of a male, this fear of causing a recurrence of back pain may in fact result in a temporary inability to achieve an erection. This fear of causing harm to the back is often unfounded. Generally, sex can be safe for the person recovering from back pain as long as the sexual activity creates minimal pain.

Often, the best way to maintain activity in this respect is to become reassured that you will not reinjure your back. For instance, the back pain sufferer should use a position that is best for him or her. Lying on the back, for instance, is frequently much more comfortable for the man than having to support the body on all fours. He may be most comfortable on his back with the female on top. A woman with a back problem, likewise, may also be more comfortable lying on her back during sex. Lying on the side or straddling the male in a seated position can also be comfortable as well as afford a certain amount of variety. In addition to these positions, there are many other ways that couples may achieve sexual fulfillment.

Remember, sex can help promote the overall recovery from back pain as well as strengthen a couple's personal relationship during a period of great stress. But as with any other activity, don't overdo it. Sex will definitely take your mind off your back pain — to the extent that it will mask pain signals to the brain. As a result, you might not feel the symptoms of back strain until the next day.

Back pain and stress

A back injury is stressful, not only because of the pain it creates, but also because of the disruption and changes that follow. Any type of change can create stress. Stress from mild change can range from being manageable to even being pleasurable. With rapid or extreme change, however, chances are the victim will experience great discomfort. It is important to remember that reacting to change in this way is a natural reaction both physically and emotionally.

There are many things we know about stress: First, we know that stress can accumulate over several years. And if this stress builds without any relief, there is likely to be some kind of physical or emotional breakdown. The symptoms of this physical, emotional, and behavioral problems include ulcers, headaches, hypertension, colitis, anger, depression, anxiety, alcohol abuse, drug abuse, eating disorders, and insomnia.

Not everyone lets stress accumulate, however. Some people can live under what would appear to be excruciating stress, yet lead comfortable lives. People who manage stress most effectively display distinctive characteristics:

- They maintain a positive attitude, looking on change as an opportunity or challenge. They focus on the future and try not to look back and whine about the past.

- They allow themselves to be involved with others, to be accountable, to feel responsible, and to share with a support group of some kind, whether it's family or friends. They are also not afraid to ask for help from professional counselors.

These same people are also good at changing personal habits to eliminate sources of self-induced stress. Here are some common sources of stress along with simple ways to eliminate them:

- Forget too easily? Write it down at the time.
- Late for work all the time? Leave home earlier.
- Traffic jams drive you nuts? Take the bus.
- Always misplace your car keys? Have a place for everything. Get organized.
- Hate having car trouble? Pay for good maintenance on your car.

When major changes occur — and the onset of back pain is a major change — it is extremely important to keep a regular routine for eating, sleeping, and exercising.

As noted throughout this book, exercise is important in managing back pain. Exercise is likewise important in managing stress. Our bodies were made for movement. Our ancestors were on the move constantly, hunting and gathering their food. They stressed their bodies by staying on the move for days at a time.

Regular aerobic activity, such as walking, biking, or swimming three times a week for 20 minutes, will help you keep stress at a distance.

Depression: The silent partner of back injury

When back pain stretches from days to weeks, or weeks to months, it begins to act as a catastrophic event in the patient's life. The term *catastrophic* is used because the event brings about a change in one's lifestyle, if even for a brief period of time. The most basic activities of daily living are generally affected, including feeding, dressing, personal hygiene, and getting from one place to another.

The usual posture one assumes while eating, for example, frequently has to be modified when one suffers from back pain. Dressing can also become much more difficult. Putting on socks, shoes, or pantyhose suddenly takes on the scope of a monumental task. Personal hygiene can seem like a chore rather than a routine. Sitting down on and rising from a commode can be an annoying source of back pain, not to mention the increase in intra-abdominal pressure that occurs during a bowel movement.

Such changes can also be accompanied by less visible ones. Following a catastrophic injury, a person can experience denial and depression. How quickly a person recovers to normal composure after denial and depression can vary.

Denial occurs in many ways. The most common is the expression of anger at not being able to do things one could previously do because of the "bloody pain" or because the "darn neck brace" is in the way. Denial in such cases is not accepting the pain or neck brace and therefore working against them instead of with them. It naturally takes a certain amount of time for a patient to accept the presence of back injury completely and begin to cope with it. Many people choose to avoid the distasteful thought of having to start back exercises because they think their back pain is somehow different. Their back pain will go away tomorrow and never return. Unfortunately, back pain usually lingers, and it almost always returns to the person who does not change his or her routine.

Depression is the most difficult stage to work through. Depression may occur because of denial. There are also many other reasons why one becomes depressed following a back injury.

The most frequent reason patients give for their depression is a feeling of inadequacy because they are not able to do even simple tasks. Being unable to do things rapidly, or with their previous skill, causes a great deal of frustration. For example, not being able to drive because of low back pain is frustrating.

In most cases, working through denial and depression requires some assistance. This may be provided by doctors, therapists, or other people who've suffered from back pain as well. Misery does love company.

Recent research has shed new light on this complex disorder. It is no longer considered a sign of weakness or a willful state, but rather a legitimate stress-related illness. Depression is now recognized as a psychosomatic ailment — one that produces observable changes in the body's biochemical or cellular structure, but which is caused or complicated by prolonged stress. The depressed patient is not unlike the person with a bleeding ulcer, someone with blinding migraines, or an executive with dangerously high blood pressure.

The brain is perhaps the most stress-sensitive of all the body parts, its chemistry extremely fragile. And it is exquisitely vulnerable to the stress of spinal injury and prolonged pain.

To maintain an even mood that accurately reflects our experiences, a delicate balance of chemicals called neurotransmitters must be maintained. Those most important are epinephrine, norepinephrine and serotonin.

If the processes involved in the manufacture, delivery, or use of these elements are upset at any stage, a chain of biochemical events is set off which does serious damage. That damage occurs in the form of a clinical depression.

Spotting depression can be difficult because the clues are not be as obvious as you might think. Feelings of profound sadness almost always occur during a depressive illness. They differ from the occasional "bad mood" in that they are deep and insatiable, yet have no observable cause.

Many patients are confused because their sorrow is so

intense despite their lives' being fairly pleasant. A nagging sense of unexplained guilt and even suicidal thoughts are also common.

Many people first notice an overwhelming fatigue, a bone-deep exhaustion that persists regardless of their workload or the amount of rest they get. This energy depletion is accompanied by a waning interest in things they normally enjoy. This can include work, hobbies, children, and sex. To their amazement (and that of their spouses), even the lustiest individuals may find that the pursuit of sex is suddenly of little importance, almost a chore.

Sleep disruption is another hallmark of depression and another example of the biochemical and physical nature of the illness. Almost all depressed individuals report a change in sleeping patterns. Some have difficulty falling asleep even though they are exhausted. Or they fall asleep quickly but awaken dozens of times throughout the long night, tossing and turning, their minds cycling endlessly through trivial topics. This is compounded for persons with back injuries because their few precious intervals of sleep are usually disrupted by pain.

Like sleep, eating is a basic human activity that is usually predictable and taken for granted. For the depressed patient, appetite can also change in unhealthy and unmanageable ways. The changes tend to occur in extremes. Either victims of depression begin to eat much more, seemingly with a bottomless hunger — or they lose all interest in food. For these reasons, depressed individuals may lose or gain a significant amount of weight. Studies show that pain patients who are depressed often develop dysfunction in both appetite and digestion.

Depression also has a symptom that complicates diagnosis in back-injured patients. It often causes an array of general aches and pains and a vague sense of "just feeling bad."

Can a person psych him- or herself out of depression? To the profound sadness of its victims, depression often will not go away through sheer will or a positive attitude. Because depression is a physical illness caused by biochemical imbalances, it cannot be wished away. Depression tends to get worse before it gets better and often requires professional treatment.

Now for the good news: depression can be treated, effectively and painlessly. Tremendous strides have been made in the two areas that are most effective in treating depression — pharmacology and psychotherapy. More depressed patients are finding relief, and faster than ever before. And today's treatments are safer, shorter, and less expensive. A combination of medication and psychotherapy (counseling) produces the fastest and most long-lasting improvement.

It is important to understand that denial and slight depression are normal responses. If you have had a recent back injury, be aware that these stages may be coming and you should be willing to discuss your feelings with others. In this way, you will be more able to accept what you are going through. Remember, it is normal to feel "down" for a period of time. It's all part of the healing process. Again, the important first step is recognizing the silent partner that often can accompany back injury. When you suspect a severe case of depression, seek professional help.

Feed your back

Most people are very conscious of maintaining their cars. They use good fuel, have tune-ups, and keep the right amount of air in the tires. Unfortunately many of us pay little attention to our bodies' fuel — our nutrition. Sadly, most Americans are overweight — which is a setup for back pain.

Also keep in mind that just as a car runs better on premium fuel, the body runs more efficiently with proper nutrition. Healing of tissue after an injury cannot occur efficiently on a junk food diet, for example. Most junk food is high in calories, high in fat, and high in sugar, with little nutritional value. Such a diet leads to weight gain and in some cases more back pain.

A simple and practical approach to good nutrition is making sure each meal contains something from each of the four main food groups. Take something from each of the following groups to help you maintain a proper diet:

Milk group — The milk group includes milk, cheese, and yogurt. Aim for two to four servings a day. Dairy products provide protein, calcium, phosphorus, and vitamin D. Selecting a low-fat type of milk is important as well.

Meat group — This group includes meat, fish, poultry, eggs, legumes, and nuts. Eat two servings a day. This category provides protein, iron, zinc, and vitamins B-6 and B-12.

Vegetable and fruit group — With four servings a day, this group will provide ample vitamins, minerals, and fiber.

Bread and cereal group — This group includes products from whole grains, enriched flour, rice and cornmeal. Four servings a day of foods from this group provide B vitamins, iron, fiber, and minerals.

Including foods from each of the four food groups will provide your body with the fuel it needs and a balance of proteins, carbohydrates, fats, vitamins, minerals, and water. The following list shows where different items fit in:

Protein — This group, which includes meat, eggs, fish, peas, beans, and dairy products, is essential for growth and repair of body tissues.

Carbohydrates — The body changes starches and sugars into glucose, which provides energy. Sources include potatoes, rice, grains, breads, pasta, beans, vegetable and fruits. Many of these foods are also high in fiber, an indigestible substance that helps move food through the body.

Fat — Fat provides energy and transports fat-soluble vitamins (vitamins A, D, E, and K). Sources of fat include vegetable oil, butter, margarine, mayonnaise, cream, peanut butter, cheese and avocados.

Water — Water is essential for transporting nutrients and eliminating wastes. Drink at least eight glasses a day.

Vitamins — Vitamins are needed for growth, maintenance, repair, and regulation of body processes. Vitamins A, D, E, and K can be stored by the body, but the others cannot be stored so daily intake is required. Vitamin A — which is needed for good vision, healthy skin, and wound healing — can be found in yellow fruits and vegetables, liver, eggs, and milk. Vitamin B — needed for utilizing carbohydrates, proteins, and fats and for proper functioning of the nervous system — is found in milk, cheese, and peas. Vitamin C helps in the formation of collagen, the connective tissue in bones, cartilage and skin. Vitamin C is very important in the healing process. It can be found in citrus fruits like oranges. Vitamin D — which helps calcium and phosphorus to be absorbed in bones — can be found in sunlight, eggs, milk, and butter. Vitamin E, which helps protect cell membranes, can can be found in vegetable oils and green leafy vegetables. Vitamin K, essential for normal blood clotting, is found in green leafy vegetables and whole grains.

Minerals — Minerals aid in the growth and structuring of bones and teeth. They also help regulate body fluid balance. Iron, for example, carries oxygen from the lungs to the cells. Iron is found in liver, oysters, prunes, beans, spinach, whole wheat, dark green vegetables, and lean red meat. Zinc aids digestion, vision, and overall growth. Fish, seafood, lean meat, eggs, fruits, and vegetables all have zinc. Calcium is necessary for continued growth and health of bones. It can be found in milk, cottage cheese, and green leafy vegetables.

Osteoporosis is a condition of decreased bone mass thought to be associated with estrogen deficiency. Lack of estrogen affects the absorption of calcium. But increasing calcium intake should be approached cautiously because too much calcium can cause complications. In osteoporosis the bones in the body begin to look like a porous sponge. As a result, bones — particularly those like the hip, wrist and spine — become brittle and fracture easily. Another contributor to osteoporosis is lack of exercise. Exercises such as walking and jogging, which stress the long bones, are best to prevent bone loss. Some people may be genetically prone to osteoporosis, but there are certain risk factors that can be controlled.

Other good tips on maintaining a healthy diet and keeping your weight in check include the following:

- Arrange to eat in one place. No meals while watching television.
- Slow your pace of eating. Chew each bite completely and put your fork down between bites.
- Serve your food on a smaller plate.
- Eat only when you are hungry, not because everyone else is eating and it is the normal time.
- Remove all fat or skin from meat or chicken.
- Broil or bake instead of frying.
- Use water-packed rather than oil-packed tuna fish.
- Avoid cream and sugar in coffee. Use skim milk.
- Avoid gravies and sauces.
- Use herbs and spices instead of butter or margarine.
- Start meals with low-calorie foods like clear soup, celery, or carrot sticks.
- Eat fresh fruits and vegetables instead of canned.
- Avoid snacking. If you must, snack on raw vegetables, broth, or gelatin.
- Exercise regularly.

Once a patient experiences an episode of back pain it is important to strengthen the musculature that surrounds the spine as well as the abdominal muscles. Patients who take care of their spines are less prone to having recurrences.

The first-aid exercises covered in this chapter are good for relieving pain and maintaining flexibility and a proper curve in the back, but they do little to strengthen muscles. That's a more intense building process.

Probably a lot of people who purchase this book rifle through to this chapter on relieving back pain. If you skipped ahead to read about first-aid remedies for your back pain, go back now and check out the earlier chapters that are specifically designed to get your back in shape. Because the best home remedy of all for back pain is to prevent it from happening in the first place.

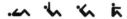

10

What can doctors do for back pain?

D o you need to see a doctor for your back pain? Maybe, maybe not. This chapter will help you decide if you need to see a doctor, and which type of doctor would be best for you. In the last chapter, we discussed home remedies for simple back pain and how for such pain a trip to the doctor might be an unnecessary expense.

Most people, for example, are surprised to learn that routine X rays show only bones. Muscles and discs, because they are soft tissue, do not show up on X ray film. Since the vast majority of simple back pain is caused by muscle strain, some spine researchers have questioned the need for X rays in treating simple back pain.

While X rays may be overused by some doctors, the fact remains that X rays are a painless and relatively inexpensive way for the physician to see inside the body and examine the structure of the spine. At the risk of oversimplifying, would you expect your mechanic to find out why your car doesn't run without ever looking under the hood? Regardless of the relative merits and limitations of X rays in diagnosing back pain, they are often helpful to the back doctor.

What X rays reveal

While X rays won't show muscles and discs, they do help the physician to rule out some serious problems — such as fractured vertebrae, vertebrae that have slipped out of alignment (spondylolisthesis), or scoliosis. X rays can also reveal narrowing of a disc space, which in turn might imply that a disc is flattening by bulging out or herniating as well as a narrowing of the spinal canal, which would imply spinal stenosis, or a problem with a facet joint, among other things.

Physicians and chiropractors primarily rely on medical histories, physical exams, and X rays to determine the cause of back pain. During the physical examination, most doctors will check the person's posture, muscle strength, sensation, and reflexes. By getting a clear description of the symptoms from the patient, and performing a careful physical exam, the doctor may begin to focus on what is causing the patient's back pain.

When back pain is caused by muscle strain, or soft tissue injury, the doctor would likely prescribe anti-inflammatories and therapy. In the case of a chiropractor, manipulation would often be performed.

Other ways to see inside the body

If your doctor is a medical doctor (M.D.), or an osteopathic doctor (D.O.), and it appears that your back problem is not related to muscle strain, the back examination may go much further and be more complex to determine the underlying cause of the pain.

A small blood sample may be drawn. A medical laboratory will then analyze the blood to determine if you have an infection or arthritis or even if there is the presence of a disease such as cancer that may be causing the symptom of back pain. Next, a urine test, called a urinalysis, may be performed to rule out a kidney problem. Low back pain is a common symptom of kidney problems, such as an infection or a kidney stone.

Thanks to technological advances over the past 10 years, there are also many new tools that can help the spine specialist see the nerves, discs, and vertebrae of the spine more clearly.

CT scans — Computed tomography uses a sophisticated X ray machine and a computer to generate X rays of the back. Unlike standard X rays, CT scans show soft tissue structures such as discs. The patient lies on a special table that passes through the center of a large scanning device. CT scans — like X rays — are painless, but they do require the person to be perfectly still while the machine scans the body.

MRI — Magnetic resonance imaging scans are an exciting advance. Unlike X rays or CT scans, which employ radiation to develop an image of the internal body, MRI uses a magnetic force along with a computer to assemble a view of the body. Like CT scans, MRI reveals discs, nerves, and bones, but in a different fashion.

EMGs — Electromyograms are often performed by a neurologist to determine if there is nerve or muscle damage. Tiny needles connected to a special instrument are used to apply pinpricks at several points along the patient's leg or arm. The slight pinpricks are more uncomfortable than they are painful. The purpose of the test is to determine if the muscle signals and nerve impulses are normal. This helps to determine if there is a pinched or damaged nerve.

Bone scans — Through a painless test, a radioactive material is injected into the bloodstream. This material then settles into the bones. Using a special instrument not unlike a Geiger counter, this radiation produces an image similar to an X ray. Bones that are undergoing rapid cell growth — as in the case of bone infection or fracture — then show up in this picture as a dense black area called a "hot spot."

Myelograms — A myelogram is a diagnostic test that also can give information regarding the relationship of the nerves to the other spinal elements such as the discs and bones. During the test, a dye is injected into the spinal canal. The patient lies on a table that is tilted so the dye slowly travels along the spine, filling the spaces surrounding the spinal nerves. The dye shows up as a white substance on X rays, while obstructions such as herniated discs or bony overgrowths causing nerve impingements are revealed as dark areas. The myelogram, while an important test, is now used less frequently since the development of CT and MRI.

Discograms — Like a myelogram, a discogram is a test that can help the surgeon decide where the pain is coming from. During a discogram, dye is injected directly into the disc. In a normal disc, the fluid would be unable to escape and would then show up as an oval on an X ray. If the disc has herniated, creating an opening in the wall of the disc, the dye is shown leaking out into an adjoining area. Because part of the nature of the test is to reproduce the pain experienced by the individual accurately, a discogram can be painful. But again, it can be a valuable test in helping to ensure that a diagnosis is correct and that any necessary surgery will be successful. The discogram plays an important role in resolving difficult cases.

Other ways M.D.'s and D.O.'s can relieve back pain

The procedures we've described help the M.D. or D.O. identify the specific nerve and disc level that is transmitting pain. Another way the physician can target the problem area is through injection techniques. By injecting a combination of cortisone and local anesthetic, not unlike what a dentist uses, into various levels in the spine, the physician can determine the specific level that is responsible for the individual's back pain as well as help treat the problem.

In an epidural steroid injection, local anesthetic and cortisone are injected into the space around the spinal nerves.

If a patient has signs of sciatica with back and leg pain, an epidural may help alleviate the patient's pain.

Facet injections are used when pain is felt to be coming from the facet joints. Injections of cortisone directly into the joint help many patients.

Trigger point injections are sometimes used to treat an area that is tender to the touch. While this area may not be the source of pain, it can act as a trigger for the onset of disabling pain.

Epidural and facet injections can be used as a diagnostic technique prior to surgery to target a problem area, or as a way to relieve pain. Sometimes pain is relieved long enough for the person to strengthen the supporting ligaments and muscles. Consequently, surgery is avoided.

M.D.'s, D.O.'s and D.C.'s: How do doctors differ?

Just as there are many different tests that can be appropriate for the range of back problems, there are different types of doctors who treat back pain. Each type of doctor differs in education, training, philosophy, and treatments used to relieve back pain.

Doctors of chiropractic (D.C.'s) — Can a chiropractor *relieve* back pain? The answer is a resounding yes. Otherwise, why would so many be in business? That is probably one of the few things that can be said without argument concerning chiropractic.

Can a chiropractor *cure* back pain? Now that is subject of great debate. In theory, chiropractors believe they relieve pain by repositioning the vertebrae so that stress on nearby nerves and joints is relieved. While many medical doctors acknowledge that chiropractic relieves pain, they don't believe any changes are permanent. In short, manipulation may relieve pain temporarily, but does it reposition anything so it stays put and there is no recurrence? According to medical research, there has yet to be a study that implies that chiropractic manipulation is a lasting treatment.

It is interesting that within the chiropractic community itself, the philosophy of chiropractic is undergoing significant evolution. At the risk of oversimplification, the traditional school of chiropractic — called "straights" — believes that many of life's problems are caused by a misalignment of the spinal vertebrae and that by forcefully realigning them, problems are cured. The second school of chiropractic thought — called "mixers" — believes that physical therapy techniques, such as ultrasound and exercise, also play a key role in the treatment of back pain.

The traditional school of chiropractic best exemplifies the tunnel vision that has made it a target of criticism by medical doctors. Critics cite that chiropractors — unlike medical doctors — do not have exposure to the vast body of knowledge related to pathology and surgery. Additionally, because they are positioned out on the fringes by themselves, they are not participants in medical research, nor are they exposed to the knowledge that is a by-product of the cross-pollination of ideas which occurs among experts in a variety of medical specialties. The perception by some medical doctors is that chiropractic is an island unto itself in an ocean of rapidly growing medical knowledge.

One of the best aspects of chiropractic is that it is a drugless treatment — mainly because D.C.'s aren't allowed to prescribe drugs. Too many times, persons with back pain are prescribed pain-relieving drugs to mask the symptoms of back pain. Over a period of years, these individuals not only retain their back problems, but they develop a serious dependency on drugs as well.

On the down side, there are chiropractors who think that spinal manipulation can cure anything. Another frequent criticism is that some chiropractors hang on to their patients indefinitely. "You're okay now, Fred, but make sure you come back next week."

It can be dangerous for any practitioner not to recog-

nize professional limitations. For instance, it can be dangerous for a chiropractor to perform manipulation on certain
back problems. Indeed, in cases involving severely herniated
discs or arthritis, chiropractic may actually worsen the problem.
Such patients should be referred to an orthopedic surgeon or
a neurosurgeon specializing in the spine.

The more current chiropractic philosophy, however,
appears to incorporate other mainstream treatments like
exercise and patient education, and as a result is beginning to
be better accepted by M.D.'s.

Doctors of osteopathy (D.O.'s) — Like the chiropractor, the osteopath incorporates an emphasis on the curative
benefits of spinal manipulation but has a formal medical
education and postgraduate training similar to that of an
M.D. Like an M.D., a D.O. can prescribe drugs.

Medical Doctors (M.D.'s) — M.D.'s, like D.O.'s, undergo a formal medical education of about four years after
completion of their college degrees. After medical school,
they often spend several more years in internship and resi-
dency before entering private practice.

The trend in medicine toward "superspecialists"

A variety of M.D.'s and D.O.'s treat back pain. The
list can include general practice physicians, physiatrists,
neurosurgeons, and orthopedic spine surgeons.

While most doctors are capable of treating simple
back strain, the challenge of treating complex back problems
is rapidly becoming a superspecialized task. Much of this
specialization is caused by rapidly changing medical technology and the volume of new research published annually.
Spine care, like sports medicine, has come a long way in the
last 10 years. And in the next five years, the field of spine
treatment will advance at an even faster pace with the
perfection of such things as percutaneous discectomy, in
which herniated discs are removed through a needle rather
than through major surgery. Similarly, the implantation of

artificial discs to replace severely degenerated discs is already being performed in Europe. Like artificial knees and hips, such new technology requires extremely specialized skills. Accordingly, it can be just plain impossible for a nonspecialist to stay well informed on advances in a particular field.

Specialization in the field of back pain can occur as a by-product of years of experience in treating only back patients, or by attending a fellowship training program that combines education with real-life experience. Most superspecialists in the field of spine care tend to be either orthopedic surgeons or neurosurgeons. Another way to measure specialization is to ask doctors if they treat anything other than the spine. A true specialist typically will focus on spine patients only. Also, ask how many and what kind of therapists the specialist has on staff. A large therapy staff can indicate that the specialist emphasizes nonsurgical treatment, or at least good rehabilitation after surgery. Having no rehabilitation staff usually leaves the surgeon with one tool in his medical arsenal: a scalpel.

The effect of superspecialization on the back patient is seen in the referral process. Some back pain sufferers are annoyed in, as they see it, being bounced from one doctor to another. In reality, their family physicians are performing a great service by providing convenient care close to patients' homes. When a patient has a complex case, the family practice physician is often the best person to assess if the patient's needs are beyond the resources available in that city and to select the appropriate superspecialist. Ultimately, the patient will be far better off in being referred to those who specialize in the spine, even if it requires a plane trip. About half of the patients who come to the Texas Back Institute, for instance, are referred by other physicians across the United States, some from as far away as Alaska.

In summary, specialization creates fantastic benefits for the patient. By choosing an area of expertise, physicians can immerse themselves in the current research so they are able to provide the most up-to-date treatments. Also, because they no longer need the generalist's equipment, they can direct all their budgets toward purchasing the latest diagnostic tools in their area of specialization, which are usually quite expensive. The same can be said for the specialist's staff. Instead of hiring therapists who know a little about everything, the specialist can hire the best in a specific field.

Other back specialists

Physical therapists — There are two aspects of physical therapy — pain relief and exercise. The passive aspects of physical therapy — heat, ultrasound, and massage — all provide relief from pain. Ultrasound is a tool that enables the therapist to radiate heat down into muscle tissue, rather than on the surface.

The second aspect of physical therapy is to move the back pain patient into exercise. There has been a lot of research in the last few years which proves that exercise is actually more beneficial than passive treatment because exercise increases endurance as well as strength and flexibility. Back pain caused by muscle spasms can be greatly relieved by getting the person to stretch out sore muscles. Exercise also increases muscle strength, which takes the load off the spine.

Physical therapy also makes an overall assessment of a patient's posture and body movements to identify any habits that may contribute to a back problem.

Most spine specialists use specialized physical therapy as one of the primary ways to resolve back pain.

Occupational therapists — Occupational therapists help patients overcome limitations and handicaps that may be imposed by injury and other health problems. Like physical therapists, occupational therapists who are specialists in back care help the patient with activities that strengthen the back and extremity muscles so the patient will be able to do more in daily living as well as on the job. This can include educating the patient as to how to lift in ways that don't strain the back, or do the activities required back on the job in less risky ways.

Exercise physiologists — As the title implies, these individuals are experts in exercise. They are trained to help individuals who have often little experience with exercise to become active and physically fit. This requires not only knowledge of the body's muscular systems, but of heart and lung systems that affect aerobic capacity as well.

Acupuncturists — Acupressure and acupuncture attempt to relieve pain in a somewhat unusual manner. As most people know, Oriental medicine is a completely different school of thought from Western medicine. The Oriental systems rely on the premise that there are energy pathways within the human body. These pathways act as highways for healing forces.

In acupuncture treatment, extremely fine needles are carefully inserted into key intersections along these pathways. It is theorized that through this needle stimulation, the acupuncturist restores the flow of healing forces to an injured area. Acupressure uses fingers instead of needles to stimulate and open these pathways.

For some people, acupressure and acupuncture can relieve a lot of symptoms. No one knows why or how, but it's hard to argue with results. Typically, acupressure and acupuncture can provide temporary, symptomatic relief for someone with a ruptured disc. But just as chiropractic can only temporarily relieve symptoms, neither acupressure nor acupuncture can repair the disc. Consequently, these types of treatments serve best as a bridge to more lasting treatments. When they are used to relieve pain long enough to get someone into an exercise program that subsequently restrengthens weak muscles, then they serve as a catalyst for therapies that bring permanent results.

What's the best treatment for back pain? As you can see, ask different people and you'll get different answers.

Although back pain is a problem experienced by 80 percent of us at some point in our lives, there is a lack of medical agreement on how the problem is best treated. Indeed, there is a vast array of professionals and paraprofessionals who treat — or attempt to treat — spine problems.

It truly is amazing that a person will agonize and shop for months for a new car, but will select a doctor in two minutes based on an ad in the yellow pages. Perhaps an even worse crime is not to ask a doctor questions about the back treatment that is prescribed. You are purchasing a service from your doctor, and you have every right to understand your treatment. If the doctor won't take the time to explain it to you, go somewhere else.

Remember, health care is as much art as it is science. Consequently, choose your back doctor carefully. It's your back and you have to live with it.

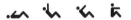

11

About back surgery

Back surgery should be the very end of the road. Each year in the United States, however, about 250,000 back surgeries are performed to remove herniated discs alone. That figure doesn't take into account other types of back surgery. Sadly, many of these back surgeries could have been avoided. Indeed, according to some experts in the field, half of all back surgeries are unnecessary.

Even under circumstances where surgery is necessary, complications can occur. Therefore, beware of a premature surgical recommendation and seek a second opinion.

The fact is, there are many treatment alternatives available before surgery need be considered. Unfortunately, when relying on a nonspecialist, the patient may have limited options, either drugs or surgery — take your pick.

We are aware of one surgeon, for example, who boasts that he provides great care at a low cost. How? He provides little or no therapy. Instead, he sends back pain sufferers home with a sheet of paper that tells them how to do their own therapy. True, as he claims, he performs surgery only on the ones who don't get better through therapy. Guess how many patients fail to cure themselves? Guess how many get back surgery? A ton.

Consider that half of the Texas Back Institute's patients are referred by other doctors — most of whom are orthopedic surgeons themselves. As a result, the clinic receives some of the worst cases of back pain imaginable. The record-setter was one unfortunate soul who had endured 24 failed back surgeries elsewhere. His spine looked like a train wreck. Yet even with such extreme cases, nearly 90 percent of patients can recover from their back problems without surgery.

To understand how far down the road back surgery should be, consider how the Texas Back Institute approaches the treatment of back pain.

Step 1: Physician exam — During the first visit, the Texas Back Institute will compile a medical history on the patient. The physician visit will involve a discussion of the person's symptoms, a neurological examination and appropriate X rays. The vast majority of patients then begin . . .

Step 2: Physical therapy — The goal of physical therapy is first to alleviate pain and then to rehabilitate the person's back so that it becomes strong again and resistant to future strain. How long a patient requires physical therapy depends on how quickly he or she responds. Many patients move quickly into a strengthening program, while other patients may require ultrasound, electrical stimulation, mobilization, or other treatments to get their pain under control. Also, if appropriate, the physical therapist may recommend . . .

Step 3: Hydrotherapy — The Texas Back Institute uses a pool and Jacuzzis to create an artificial weightlessness for the patient. In short, activities that would normally be too painful to do — such as walking — become tolerable in water. Not only does the water provide the therapeutic effect of relieving pain, it helps get a person active and ready for . . .

Step 4: Extensive exercise — Exercise is perhaps the foundation of any effective back treatment because it is one of the few treatments that has a permanent effect — if the person accepts it into his or her own daily routine. In addition to a customized exercise program, the patient can benefit from additional instruction in the form of a . . .

Step 5: Back School — Since lifestyle is a major contributing factor to back pain, the Texas Back Institute focuses on lifestyle changes that enable the individual to assume responsibility for his or her own health. Through the Back School, individuals learn how to lift, push, pull, sit, and stand in ways that won't strain the back. The Back School covers the anatomy of the spine, first aid for back injury, exercises that relieve back pain, controlling pain without drugs, body mechanics, biofeedback, and relaxation techniques. If patients need more in-depth help regarding pain management, they proceed to . . .

Step 6: Biofeedback — Pain is a signal to the brain. And just like an electronic signal, it can be interrupted. It can be tempting to rely on drugs to interrupt this pain signal. For those people with ongoing back pain, however, drug use can lead to its own set of problems. There are ways to interrupt the pain signal in ways that don't involve drugs, however. Transcutaneous Electrical Nerve Stimulation (TENS) units, for one, can be used to temporarily "short-circuit" back pain. Over the past few years, TENS units have become popular among professional athletes for accelerated rehabilitation of injured arms and legs. Doctors aren't sure why electrical stimulation provides pain relief, but some theorize that the intermittent current causes the brain to release endorphins, the body's own chemical painkiller.

Another technique that can be used is biofeedback. It's been proven medically that the mind can lower heart rate and blood pressure. Through training, the back pain sufferer can reduce back pain by distracting the mind from the pain signal. Many people are so consumed by pain that their lives aren't fun anymore. In addition to biofeedback techniques, patients are encouraged to explore activities that can keep their minds off their back pain. Photography, fishing, and painting are just a few nonphysical ways to involve and distract the mind from pain. Another pain management treatment is . . .

Step 7: Injection techniques — As noted in the last chapter, some types of pain can be eliminated by injecting cortisone into a particular point in the back. The relief can last from weeks to years. In many cases, such injections succeed in relieving pain long enough for the injury to heal and for the person to recondition and strengthen the supporting muscles in the back. Finally, beyond pain management techniques, patients may proceed to . . .

Step 8: Diagnostic tests — Other tests like CT, MRI, discograms, and myelograms can help diagnose the cause of a person's back pain and indicate if surgery is necessary.

If surgery is necessary

Only after all these steps have been exhausted should surgery be considered a viable alternative. If you feel that surgery has been recommended hastily for you, explore a second opinion from another specialist.

Here is an overview of some common back and neck surgeries and what they are intended to accomplish. Generally, the surgeon tries either to stabilize elements in the spine, or to decompress elements such as discs which may be pinching nearby nerves. Unless otherwise noted, the patient is under general anesthesia. Traditional back surgery typically requires hospitalization for several days and at least a month for recovery.

Discectomy — A discectomy is intended to remove that part of a badly herniated disc which is pressing on nearby nerves. Through the procedure, the surgeon removes a portion of the herniated disc to relieve pressure on nerves. It is important to remember that not all of the disc is removed in this procedure. A large portion of the outer rim of the disc remains and continues to act as a shock absorber between the vertebrae.

Fusion — The purpose of a surgical fusion is to stabilize vertebrae that are inherently unstable or have become unstable because of a degenerative disc or badly worn facet joint. Using bone obtained from the patient's pelvis or from a bone bank, the surgeon grafts bone alongside two vertebrae. Over time, the bone usually heals together, forming a stable bridge between the two levels.

Foramenotomy — The purpose of a foramenotomy is to relieve the irritation on spinal nerves caused by spinal stenosis. Just as a tight ring can cause a finger to swell painfully, there are small openings in the vertebrae, called foramen, that provide a passageway for the spinal nerves. Over time, these openings can become restrictive, causing the nerve to swell and inflame. Through a foramenotomy, the surgeon carefully shaves bone around the foramen to free up space for the nerve and decrease inflammation. In a sense, the procedure is like having your jeweler enlarge your ring so your finger is no longer crimped and blood can circulate freely.

Rhizotomy — Through a rhizotomy, the surgeon attempts to relieve a person's facet joint pain by interrupting, or cutting, the nerves of the vertebral facet joint. The result is that the facet joint loses its ability to transmit pain to the brain.

Percutaneous discectomy — Percutaneous discectomy is one of the latest advances in spine surgery. Using a tiny probe, the spine surgeon is able to remove portions of a herniated disc through an incision that can afterward be covered with a Band-Aid. As in a traditional discectomy, not all the disc is removed, just enough to relieve the pressure on irritated nerves. The Texas Back Institute was one of several clinical sites across the nation which evaluated the tool when it was introduced in 1986. Unlike traditional spine surgery, the procedure is done under local anesthesia, and the patient can return home right afterward or after an overnight observation in the hospital. The patient can often resume activity in as little as a week. Unfortunately, the procedure is limited to only those disc herniations that can be reached by the probe.

Surgery to correct scoliosis — As noted in Chapter 2, scoliosis first appears in adolescence, when youngsters go through the growth spurt. If the spinal curvature is detected early, new types of braces can be used to help control and correct the curve. When this is not possible, many times the spine can and should be straightened surgically.

The best corrective procedures are those done at a young age, when the spine is more flexible and better able to tolerate the stress of surgical straightening. As we get older, the spine becomes less flexible and more brittle. In fact, few orthopedic surgeons attempt adult scoliosis surgery because of the expertise required.

Thanks to advances in surgical instrumentation, such as the Cotrel-Dubousset rods, surgeons are able to untwist and straighten the spine in ways never before possible. Cotrel-Dubousset rods were invented in France and have been available for use in the United States since 1985. Another system of surgical fixation tools, called Harrington rods, has been in use since 1962. While both fixation systems attempt to straighten the curve by using two rods on either side of the spinal column, the principles used are quite different.

With Harrington rods, the scoliosis surgeon has only two hooks, top and bottom, to secure to the vertebrae. Instead of just two hooks, Cotrel-Dubousset rods employ several hooks that attach to several vertebrae at various levels in the spine. This helps to secure the rods in place better and allows for a different method of straightening. Unlike Harrington rods, which force the twisted spine into a more upright position, Cotrel-Dubousset rods attempt to undo what Mother Nature did wrong by actually untwisting the corkscrew-like curve. Harrington rods, conversely, cannot rotate the vertebrae because there are only two points of fixation. As a result, the curve is corrected not by untwisting a twisted spine, but by stretching out the curve in the spine. That in itself carries with it some risks because the spinal cord may be stretched and damaged. The worst consequence of pushing such a system too far can be permanent paralysis.

When it comes to any kind of back surgery, invest the time and energy to locate a surgeon or clinic that specializes in spine care. In many cases, you may find that surgery can be avoided altogether. But if not, the risks will be diminished and the outcome will more likely be successful.

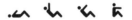

12

Questions we've been asked

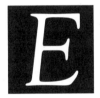ach year, the Texas Back Institute's Back Pain Hotline handles more than 5,000 calls and letters from individuals with back pain. By now, the nurses have heard virtually every possible question 10 times over. If you have back pain, you may have wondered about the following questions, too.

Questions about daily activities

How long should I sit?

Doing anything that puts the spine in a static position, that is, a position where it is denied movement, creates a great degree of stress and heightens the risk of back strain. People who sit at computer terminals for long periods of time without getting up and walking around often suffer from back, and especially neck, pain.

At least once an hour, you should stand, walk around,

bend, arch backward slightly, and twist — all to create movement in the back and free up the muscles and joints. Doing so
at regular intervals will lengthen the amount of time you can
sit comfortably.

Having a properly designed chair, or an orthopedic
insert, will also support the spine and make for more comfortable sitting. If sitting is part of your job, buy a good chair. It
may be one of the best tools you can have. (See Chapter 8 for
more information.)

How can I counteract the stress from sitting?

Utilize back or neck supports in sitting and keep your
back relatively straight. In short, don't slouch. It may feel
comfortable at the time, but it puts an extreme load on your
spine. Instead, belly up to the table and get close to your work.
Having to lean over and reach puts additional weight and
strain on your back. Also, keep your knees slightly higher
than your hips. This will encourage alignment of the spine
and prevent you from getting into a slouched position.

Is there a good way to get in and out of a chair without discomfort?

Slide to the edge of the chair using your armrest. Use
leg power as you inhale to come to a standing position. Make
sure you don't hold your breath, which may unnecessarily
tense your arms. To sit back down, touch the back of your
knees to the chair and keep your feet shoulder width apart.
Exhale as you sit at the edge of the chair, then scoot backward.

*I hate standing, but it's a big part of my job. Is there a comfortable
way to do it?*

Nurses, sales clerks, toll booth operators, factory
workers — you name it. So many jobs require people to be on
their feet for nine hours straight. The worst possible job is one
that does not allow the person to walk around, requiring that
he or she stay standing at a work station or counter.

Prolonged standing increases the spinal curvature,

which in turn results in the compression of facet joints. One way to lessen the strain on the body's natural curves is to stand tall, feet flat on the ground, with equal weight on both.

If you have to stand for long periods, prop one foot on a small stool or telephone book to decrease stress in the low back. Alternate with the other foot. When washing dishes, open the cabinet below the sink and let one foot rest on the ledge.

Then every half hour, bend over and touch your toes with your knees slightly bent. This will help loosen and unbind the muscles, ligaments, and joints. Remember what happened to the Tin Man in *The Wizard of Oz?* The spine likes to be mobile — that's the only way it can create its own internal lubricant. Like the Tin Man, when it stops moving for long periods, it freezes up.

Should I sleep on my back or on my stomach or side?

The one time of the day during which the spine can totally relax and recharge its muscles and ligaments for the day ahead is when we are asleep.

The best of all positions is to lie on your back with a small pillow tucked underneath the knees. This position completely unloads the spine and restores a natural curve to the back.

An alternate position is to lie on your side with a pillow between your knees.

Lying face down can put stress on the back. If you like sleeping on your stomach, place a soft, flat pillow under your stomach. This will help eliminate some of the arch that would otherwise occur.

Is a firm mattress better for a bad back? Are waterbeds good for the back?

It's important to sleep on a good mattress with good back support. Years ago, waterbeds were mushy and provided little support for the back. And generally, physicians at the

Texas Back Institute cautioned patients against them. Times have changed. Now you can buy waterbeds that allow you to adjust the firmness and the temperature of the water.

Still, waterbeds are definitely not for everybody. On the other side, too many doctors have made sleep uncomfortable by overgeneralizing and recommending firm mattresses for everybody. The fact is, everybody is built differently.

Generally speaking, any mattress that helps you sleep comfortably, so you wake up refreshed, is good for you. For some people, that may mean sleeping on a mattress that feels like a rock. But others, especially those with large buttocks, find that a firm mattress doesn't conform to their body curves. As a result, it's uncomfortable.

The best medical advice on mattresses is to "test-drive" a mattress to find one that is comfortable for you. Try going to different hotels and see how you sleep. Then check out the mattress brand and stiffness, accordingly. Most importantly, if you have a mattress that is uncomfortable for you, get rid of it.

Is there an easy way to get out of bed when you have back pain? What is the logrolling technique?

Sometimes getting in and out of your bed is hard when you're experiencing back pain. Logrolling is getting in and out of bed by first rolling over to the side of the bed and lowering your feet to the ground. This makes it easier to sit up on the edge of the bed and then stand.

Here's how you do it: lying on your back in bed, roll over on your side toward the edge of the bed, making sure that your shoulders and hips move together. Don't twist. Once on your side facing outward at the edge of the bed, gently bring your knees up until your feet dangle off the edge of the bed. From that position, use your hands and elbow to push up against the bed, while at the same time you use the weight of your legs as a counterbalance to help you to sit up on the edge of the bed. From that position, just stand up.

The purpose of the logrolling technique is to minimize the twisting of the body and to use arm strength rather than sore trunk muscles to lift yourself up and out of bed.

What is the best back support?

There are many types of back support to choose from. It all depends on where you need to use it. A car back support, for example, may be different from a support for an office chair. Some of the more common back supports are Back Friend, Obus Form, Relax-a-bac, and Spinebac. Again, the purpose of a back support is to maintain the natural lordotic curve or enhance the midposition. Choose the right one for you.

Do you recommend using a lifting belt when working out in the gym or when heavy lifting is required on the job?

For years, weight lifters have used heavy leather belts to support their backs during their workouts. Today, lifting belts are available in a variety of designs. Similarly, there are lightweight plastic and fabric weaves that provide equal support and better comfort than a stiff leather lifting belt.

The nonprofit Texas Back Institute Research Foundation is studying the effectiveness of lifting belts in reducing back injury. It appears that weight belts help some individuals lift slightly heavier weights. The theory is that the belt supports the abdominal muscles, which play a key role in lifting. Another theory, however, holds that the belt acts as a crutch and prevents the back from strengthening itself fully through continual lifting.

One thing is for sure, wearing a weight belt reminds the person to protect the back. This may then cause the person to use proper body mechanics and use the legs and other supporting muscles in the lift.

Without doubt, it appears that weight belts help the back in some way. How weight belts actually work, and if they can reduce lifting injuries, is something that needs more formal study. If a weight belt feels good to you, makes you feel more confident, and reminds you that you need to be careful lifting, then it makes sense to use one.

How can long plane trips be made more comfortable for someone with back pain?

Fly first class or business class if possible. The seats are wider and more comfortable. It is also helpful to raise your feet up on an briefcase or carry-on bag under the seat in front of you. Lastly, ask for a pillow to place behind your back to improve lumbar support.

Questions about drugs

What are the most commonly used over-the-counter drugs for back pain?

Of all the nonprescription drugs, acetaminophen, aspirin and the ibuprofen products like Advil, Nuprin, and Medipren have become the most commonly used medications by people suffering from back pain.

How do they work?

Acetaminophen, which is in Tylenol and Datril, for example, acts as an analgesic and antipyretic to reduce pain and fever. Essentially, acetaminophen has the least anti-inflammatory effect, while ibuprofen has more anti-inflammatory effect but less analgesic effect. And aspirin is somewhere in the middle.

If you were to recommend an over-the-counter medication for simple back pain, what would it be?

Generally, for most musculoskeletal back pain, that is, pain emanating from the muscles, tissues, ligaments, and bones, there is going to be some inflammation. Therefore, to aid the healing process, and indirectly relieve the pain, I'd recommend aspirin or any of the ibuprofen products.

It seems that many new drugs are available over the counter. Why is that?

In the past, a person needed a prescription for any of the ibuprofen products, but now the U.S. Food and Drug Administration has found that in the low doses that are packaged for over-the-counter sales, they are really very safe.

How do over-the-counter doses compare with those of prescription drugs?

The prescription versions of ibuprofen, like Motrin, come in 400, 600, and 800 milligram doses, while the over-the-counter versions are typically only 200 milligrams. The doctor might prescribe other anti-inflammatory prescription-only drugs like Naprosyn, Indocin, or Feldene, which are chemically different from ibuprofen.

What are the negative side effects of the favorite over-the-counter back drugs?

Overdosing on an acetaminophen product, like Tylenol, can have a side effect on a person's liver. In extreme cases, it can cause irreversible liver damage. Overdosing on aspirin can, in the worst case, cause a coma. A more common side effect of too much aspirin is that some people develop stomach ulcers. Similarly, overdosing on ibuprofen can also cause gastric problems.

Is there any benefit in buying brand-name aspirin or acetaminophen versus generic?

Not really. But there are subtle differences.

The therapeutic effect of aspirin is the same whether it is Bayer, Bufferin, Excedrin, or whatever. But some aspirin tablets — like the brands Ecotrin or Encaprin — are enteric-coated to prevent the irritation that can occur in the stomach with some people. This coating can help the pills to withstand the acids in the stomach so they can be broken down later by the enzymes in the intestines.

Using a different approach, Bufferin and Ascriptin, for example, contain ingredients like Maalox to make the aspirin less acidic and lessen stomach irritation. But's that's not as proven as the enteric-coating approach.

In short, those people who complain that their stomachs hurt 10 minutes after taking aspirin, should consider taking an enteric-coated aspirin. And if such symptoms persist, stop and consult a doctor.

What about buying the "extra-strength" versions of aspirin or acetaminophen?

You're really just buying higher doses. The common dose of regular Tylenol, for example, is 325 milligrams. The extra-strength dose is 500 milligrams.

Generally, with medicine, always try to take the lowest dose that works. The higher the dose, the greater the side effects.

Is there any danger to relying on over-the-counter medicine to treat back pain?

Yes. The danger is that you could be ignoring important signals from your body. Pain medicine, for instance, has no effect on numbness or muscle weakness. You need to pay attention to those signs.

Questions about treatments

What about non-drug pain relief? What other first-aid remedies can a person use immediately after a back injury? Should a person apply ice or heat to the back?

Remember this rule: ice first for 48, then heat.

There is definitive research that proves that ice slows the swelling and inflammation that occur after injury. After 48 hours, ice has lost its effect. Using heat thereafter aids the healing process by increasing circulation and relaxing muscle spasms. But the research on the benefits of heat is less conclusive. Ice we know is beneficial. Heat we're not so sure about.

What about home massage?

For simple muscle-related back strain that involves the upper back or neck, massage may be beneficial. Massage on the low back may provide some temporary relief as well.

Is there an artificial disc that can be used to replace my damaged disc?

Spine researchers are actively trying to develop an artificial disc that can replace badly deteriorated discs. None is available for wide-scale use in the United States at this time, but the future does indeed look bright.

Are there any back pain symptoms or signals that would tell a person that he or she should see a doctor, rather than rely on home remedies?

Yes. If you find that you're doubling up on your Advil or Nuprin, you need to tell your doctor.

Foot drop, where a person drags a foot because his or her leg muscles cannot raise the toes, is a sign of a serious neurological problem such as nerve impingement or a ruptured disc. Similarly, loss of bowel or bladder control is a serious danger signal. A person with either symptom should go immediately to a spine specialist or to a hospital emergency room. If you ignore signals like this, the loss of muscular control could become permanent.

Radicular pain, which radiates down an arm or leg, implies that a nerve is being pinched, perhaps from a bulging or ruptured disc. It too is a signal to see a spine specialist.

Will surgery resolve my back problem?

Even if surgery is necessary, it alone will not ensure the

future health of your back. You will need a coordinated rehabilitation program that will strengthen your back, improve its flexibility, and condition you aerobically. You will also need to learn proper body mechanics to lessen the risk of reinjury.

What will replace my disc if it is removed surgically?

Only the protruding part of the disc is actually removed from the area of the spinal canal where it doesn't belong. The undiseased part of the disc remains in place and continues to act as a shock absorber for your spine.

Questions about back doctors

Assuming a person has exhausted all home remedies and visits a back specialist, what is the examination like? What is the doctor looking for?

X rays are taken to see if there are any bone tumors, acute emergent situations, or congenital defects that have been hidden up until now.

While simple X rays would not reveal a herniated disc, they can show signs that might indicate a disc problem.

How does a doctor determine if a person's pain is from a disc problem?

Disc herniations would appear on a CT scan, magnetic resonance imaging or a myelogram, so those tests might be ordered later on.

When should I get a second opinion?

If your insurance company asks you, or if you have any doubts about a recommended treatment.

Most good doctors have no objections to a patient's getting a second opinion. If your doctor does object, maybe he or she is not the right doctor for you.

Insurance companies have good reason to recommend second opinions, by the way. They've documented a phenomenon called the "sentinel effect." While second opinions often confirm the first specialist, insurance companies have noted that the total number of surgeries does indeed go down over time. They theorize that doctors, knowing that their advice will be reviewed by a second doctor, become more prudent with their surgical recommendations.

What does informed consent mean?

Informed consent means the doctor or his staff has explained the procedures that you are about to receive and you understand the explanation. If you have any questions about any type of treatment you are about to receive, be sure to ask, and ask again, until everything is clear to you.

How does a person find a good back doctor?

Personal recommendation from a friend is sometimes a good place to start. But don't stop there. Next, do your own homework. Find out about the doctor's education, experience and credentials.

Medical doctors, that is M.D.'s, have boards of specialization which provide certification of advanced expertise in various specialties. This board certification is based on written and oral exams as well as experience. Ask if your doctor is board certified. A variety of medical specialists address back problems, including orthopedic surgeons, neurosurgeons, physiatrists and occupational medicine physicians. Many of these specialties provide fellowship training, the most advanced type of training available. You might ask if your doctor is fellowship trained in the field of spine care.

Perhaps the best possible way to find a good back doctor is to select someone who treats only back patients. Simply put, specialization breeds excellence. Another good indicator is that the physician or clinic has therapy and exercise protocols. Remember, surgery should be the last alternative. Make sure you select a doctor who offers plenty of other alternatives as well.

How does chiropractic provide pain relief?

Chiropractic uses manipulation of the spine, in addition to passive physical therapy techniques such as applying heat and ultrasound to achieve relief of pain. For muscle-related back pain, chiropractic can be an effective therapy.

A lot of patients are referred by chiropractors to the Texas Back Institute when they have problems that are not responding to chiropractic.

There are certain cases where chiropractic or osteopathic manipulation can be dangerous — such as in a severely herniated disc, or when there is a spine tumor.

Ask your chiropractor how he or she treats back pain patients. Progressive chiropractors focus on more than just temporarily relieving pain with manipulation and heat. Look for a chiropractor who emphasizes exercise in his or her treatment program.

How do acupressure and acupuncture relieve pain?

For some people, acupressure or acupuncture can relieve a lot of symptoms. No one knows why or how, but it's hard to argue with results. Like chiropractic, acupressure or acupuncture can provide temporary, symptomatic relief for someone with a ruptured disc. But it doesn't fix the disc or strengthen the muscles that surround and protect it.

What about physical therapy?

The passive aspects of physical therapy — heat, ultrasound, massage — all provide relief of pain. The active aspect of physical therapy, however, is exercise. A lot of research in the last few years shows that exercise is actually more beneficial than the passive treatments.

But doesn't exercise sound painful to persons with back pain?

    True. But exercise is the best way to centralize their pain from a broad area to a localized area, reduce pain, accelerate the healing process, and lastly prevent the injury from happening again. And those are the the kinds of results we at the Texas Back Institute are after.

13

Troubleshooting

Half of all back surgeries performed in the United States are unnecessary. How can you make sure that you don't become a statistic? (1) If you have a serious back problem, go to a back specialist — someone who treats only backs; (2) make sure that the specialist has lots of therapists; and (3) if surgery is recommended, be sure to get a second opinion.

When back pain strikes, it's natural to think the worst. But remember: 80 percent of back pain is simple muscle strain. This chapter may help you identify the source of your pain. No book can diagnose a problem, however. Consequently, if your pain doesn't go away after three days, be safe and see a back doctor.

Symptom	Possible causes	Possible treatment
Sharp, piercing pain limited to a small area in the back	• Muscle strain • Ligament strain • Disc injury • Joint injury	• Medication to reduce swelling • Ice for 48 hours to reduce swelling, then heat to encourage healing • Therapy, which could include pain-relief methods such as ice, heat, and ultrasound. Exercise to improve range of motion and circulation. Strengthening program to recondition muscles and prevent a recurrence of pain
Pain in low back when extending, bending backward	• Joint inflammation • Slippage of one vertebra on another	• Mild medication to reduce swelling • Use of corset or lifting belt when participating in exercise or work
Pain in low back when flexing, bending forward	• Muscle or ligament strain • Poor physical condition • Facet syndrome • Possible disc problem	• Medication to reduce swelling • Reconditioning program, including physical therapy for flexibility and muscle balancing, weight loss, etc.
Low back pain occurring in the last few months of pregnancy	• Extra weight is pulling low back vertebrae forward, causing discomfort to muscles and ligaments	• Avoiding activity that stresses the back until after baby is delivered • With doctor's approval, a water exercise program • After delivery, reconditioning and strengthening the back with a home or gym exercise program
Back or leg pain or pain behind the hip area which occurs only after sitting for long periods, and especially after driving for long periods	• Sciatic nerve, which runs from the back down into the leg, is becoming irritated from from too much sitting	• Reducing the time spent sitting, or taking several breaks to walk around. If this is not possible, buying an orthopedically designed chair, car seat, or seat insert to reduce pressure on sciatic nerve • Exercise program
Pain that begins in upper back and extends into shoulder, but not to elbow	• Bulging or herniated disc that is irritating a nerve root • Neck strain • Arthritis of cervical spine	• Medication to reduce swelling • Use of cervical collar • Exercise to improve range of motion and circulation
Pain limited to the neck area	• Muscle strain • Ligament strain • Arthritis	• Medication to reduce inflammation • Soft cervical collar • Exercise program to strengthen and recondition muscles

Symptom	Possible causes	Possible treatment
Pain in the arm	• *Bulging or herniated disc* • *Arthritis* • *Degenerative disc disease* • *Other non-spine causes*	• *Medication to reduce swelling around nerve* • *Soft cervical collar* • *Mild exercise program to improve range of motion and circulation* • *If all corrective actions fail, surgery may be needed to remove the herniated disc or stabilize vertebrae*
Pain that begins in upper back, and extends down the arm past the elbow	• *Bulging or herniated disc is irritating a nerve root* • *Narrowing of openings where nerves exit vertebrae, either from injury or arthritis*	• *Medications to reduce swelling* • *Cervical collar or cervical traction* • *Mild exercise program to improve range of motion and circulation* • *If conservative treatment is not successful, surgery may be needed to relieve pressure on nerves*
Foot drop. When walking, front of foot drags, muscles unable to raise the front part of the foot	• *Herniated disc at L4-L5* • *Severe spinal stenosis*	• *Seek help from orthopedic surgeon or neurosurgeon*
Loss of bowel or bladder control. Inability to control urination	• *Impingement of nerve roots, usually from herniated disc*	• *Immediately see an orthopedic surgeon or neurgosurgeon. If that is not possible, go to a hospital emergency room. Consider this a serious emergency. If not treated promptly, there could be permanent nerve and muscle damage*
Pain in the leg	• *Spinal stenosis* • *Degenerative disc disease* • *Herniated or bulging disc*	• *Short-term bed rest* • *Medication to reduce swelling* • *Mild exercise program to improve range of motion, circulation and strength* • *Possible surgery*
Posture gradually worsening, with a noticeable hump appearing in the upper back or with alignment of back becoming crooked	• *Osteoporosis. Bones are becoming porous and brittle* • *Scoliosos. Spine may be curving. Curvature usually appears in adolescent years*	• *See an orthopedic surgeon. If the problem is osteoporosis, dietary supplements may be recommended, as well as other treatment. If the problem is scoliosis, braces may be recommended. Surgery may be needed to correct certain cases and prevent life-threatening complications*

Acknowledgments

Paula Gilbert,
Physical Therapist,
Texas Back Institute

Billy Glisan,
Exercise Physiologist,
Texas Back Institute

Suggested Reading

Alter, Judy. *Stretch and Strengthen*. Boston: Houghton Mifflin Co., 1986.

Bailey, Covert. *Fit or Fat?* Boston: Houghton Mifflin Co., 1977, 1978.

Hall, M.D., Hamilton. *The Back Doctor*. New York: Berkley Books 1980.

Hogan, Ben. *Five Lessons — The Modern Fundamentals of Golf*. New York: Simon & Schuster, Inc.

Noble, Elizabeth. *Essential Exercises for the Childbearing Year*. 3d ed., rev. Boston: Houghton Mifflin Co., 1988.

Index